THE
COOL
FACTOR

THE COOL FACTOR

A Guide to Achieving Effortless
Style, with Secrets from the
Women Who Have It

ANDREA LINETT
Photographs by Michael Waring

ARTISAN
NEW YORK

Library of Congress Cataloging-in-Publication Data
Linett, Andrea, author.
    The cool factor / Andrea Linett.
        pages cm
    Includes index.
    ISBN 978-1-57965-648-5
    1. Fashion. 2. Women's clothing. I. Title.
    TT507.L5269 2016
    746.9'2—dc23   20150342420

Design by Naomi Mizusaki, Supermarket

Artisan books are available at special discounts
when purchased in bulk for premiums and sales
promotions as well as for fund-raising or educational
use. Special editions or book excerpts also can be
created to specification. For details, contact the
Special Sales Director at the address below, or send
an e-mail to specialmarkets@workman.com.

Published by Artisan
A division of Workman Publishing Company, Inc.
225 Varick Street
New York, NY 10014-4381
artisanbooks.com

Published simultaneously in Canada by
Thomas Allen & Son, Limited

Printed in China
First printing, March 2016

10 9 8 7 6 5 4 3 2 1

For my dad, Gene Linett, who was always the coolest-dressed cat on the block

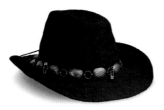

Contents

Introduction

Cool is such a funny word. Like *pretty* or *smart,* the meaning—and the designation—is entirely subjective. Some might consider it to be an intimidating description, or even an immature one, like something you would call the Fonz or a rock star of the moment. But to me, cool, when pertaining to style, means personalization and effortlessness. (No one looks cool blatantly copying someone else or trying too hard.)

And cool is also about *real* style, something I was obsessed with even when I worked at high-end women's magazines covering designer fashion. Although my job was to get super excited about what was on the runways (and sometimes I did), I confess that nothing was more thrilling than checking out the actual working women filing into the venues. The best were the European editors—French and Italian— looking unbelievably cool and sexily disheveled. Unlike their American counterparts, who usually were all dressed identically, no two women looked alike, and each had a distinct aesthetic. *That* was where the true inspiration was!

I've been on a quest to demystify that kind of easy, cool style since I was a kid. I always knew there was a book in there somewhere, decoding the elements of cool for a broader audience. But it wasn't until a Maria Cornejo trunk show at Bird, the cult women's clothing store in Brooklyn, that the concept truly took shape. My plan for the evening was simply to go grab a glass of wine and order a few cute fall pieces (which I did). But, much to my delight, the event proved a veritable master class in real-woman style inspiration. Walking in, I found myself surrounded by cool women of every age, all perfectly put together in that effortless, un-fashion-y, super-stylish way that I so admire. It was almost too much to take in.

And I loved that none of them were "kids": their ages ranged from late thirties to fifty and over. Which, when I thought about it, made perfect sense. These women had been around the fashion block and had tried everything over the years, and thus they knew what *truly* worked for them.

I had the sudden urge to round everyone up, photograph them, and have them divulge how they put themselves together. So, around six months later, that's exactly what I did. Now, imagine the coolest women you know dragging big rolling suitcases—filled with their favorite pieces—into a photo studio. It was a crazy fashion-inspiration party that unfolded over the course of four days. Everyone checked out each other's stuff, compared notes, and did a bit of mental shopping and personal styling.

In converting a photo shoot into text, I set out to write an atypical fashion book. In line with my own personal style, I strove to keep it somewhat "untucked" and casual yet with an underlying meticulousness that comes from having a finely honed eye. Most style books will tell you what *not* to do, and how to look professional or presentable by following hard-and-fast rules made up by "fashion" people. In contrast, this book talks about dressing for everyday scenarios, and reveals tricks to make you feel more special. My goal is to arm you with ideas that will help you find and build on your *own* personal style—to show you how to dress like a cool, *real* woman. Here, you will find tons of unconventional tips for what to look for when shopping, and how to make the most of the clothes already in your closet. Being cool doesn't involve wearing certain labels, but rather knowing what works for you—even if it's a piece from a dorky line.

Cool is about *real* style, something I was obsessed with even when I worked at high-end women's magazines covering designer fashion.

I never read visual books in a linear fashion, and I don't expect you to, either. I usually flip through, find something that catches my eye, and then dive a bit deeper into that section, often dog-earing my favorite pages. The sections and spreads in this book are designed to be digested modularly, and you might be surprised at the chapter topics. Some are super specific (a whole section on the miracle fabric that is denim!), while others are more practical (how *do* you wear leather, anyway?).

I have always had a secret mental "library" of inspiration to tap into when shopping or getting dressed: an arsenal of cool women—my personal icons, if you will. These are the ones who will be eternally cool, no matter their age. I think of Jane Birkin and Kate Moss when I want to be rock 'n' roll sexy, and Lauren Hutton and Charlotte Gainsbourg when I'm feeling more classic-cool. And then there are all the real women I see around every day who provide me with endless ideas about how I want to look and present myself.

I could have hired professional models to illustrate the styling points, but that would have been counterintuitive, since the thrill is in decoding how the real women I know dress so cool. So who better to show us? Allow me to introduce you to the "models"—style role models, all—thirty-three women ranging in age from mid-twenties to mid-seventies. Meet them, see which ones you relate to, and then follow them through the book. Maybe take rocker jewelry inspiration from one and classic styling from another. In other words, I don't suggest that you follow one woman's style to a T. Pick and choose from each to come up with your own look; that's the fun of it!

I want to thank each of them for taking time out of their busy schedules to show up, spend the day with me, share their tips and tricks, and break it all down for us without holding back any secrets—because *that's* really, really cool.

Here, you will find tons of unconventional tips for what to look for when shopping, and how to make the most of the clothes already in your closet.

Meet the Models

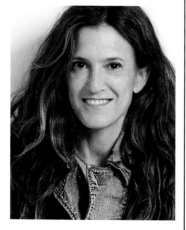

ANDREA LINETT, creative director

Self-described style: I always say "untucked glamour," with the emphasis on "untucked." I love good clothes and fun shapes, but somehow I never look too put together—and I feel most comfortable that way.

Anne Johnston Albert, creative director and illustrator

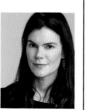

Why: We've been best friends since tenth grade, and she is my go-to style person whenever I need an opinion. We've collaborated on many projects, most recently our capsule collection, JOLIE/Laide.

Self-described style: "Undone classic. I stick to and appreciate tailored, timeless pieces, but I pair them with worn-in or unfussy items."

Jennifer Alfano, fashion writer and jewelry designer

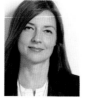

Why: We worked together at *Harper's Bazaar*, and she was always the chicest girl in the room.

Self-described style: "Timeless, modernist, and tailored. Nothing too girlie, except for the occasional printed silk dress."

Anna Bakst, president, Michael Kors Accessories

Why: Anna is the coolest! She just knows how to rock a classic in a really laid-back and sexy way.

Self-described style: "Casual. There's nothing better than wearing worn-in jeans with a white T-shirt, flip-flops, and sunglasses. In fact, I've become more casual as I've gotten older."

Christene Barberich, editor in chief, Refinery29

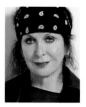

Why: Christene knows the right mix: her cool hair, makeup, and interesting combos of vintage and new pieces are always fun to look at. And she never follows trends.

Self-described style: "I love the extreme elegance of minimalism, but I'm also helplessly drawn to pairing unsavory colors and patterns: that ugly-pretty Prada gene in me cannot be denied."

Bibi Cornejo Borthwick, photographer (and daughter of Maria Cornejo)

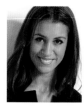

Why: She always looks effortless, whether she's wearing one of her mom's cool designs or just her favorite jeans and a vintage army jacket.

Self-described style: "I love being timeless and comfortable at all times!"

Maria Cornejo, fashion designer

Why: If I could afford to fill an entire closet with her designs, I would. She is the epitome of easy cool.

Self-described style: "Feminine androgyny; I'm not a girlie-girl. And I'm less edgy than I used to be."

Linda Dresner, boutique owner

Why: Linda is a legend. Any woman who can rock an Axl Rose–style head bandana (her signature) with a major avant-garde designer like Rei Kawakubo is cool in my book.

Self-described style: "I wear a combination of old Comme des Garçons, Jean Muir, Yohji Yamamoto, and Martin Margiela with new pieces mixed in."

Laura Ferrara, stylist and farmer

Why: Every time I see her on the street, I wish I had on exactly what she is wearing—always a hip mix of classics with slightly edgier pieces. And her thick mane of hair is enviable.

Self-described style: "Masculine with bohemian details. No makeup and low maintenance. And I hate wearing nail polish!"

Mimi Fisher, stylist

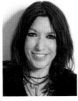

Why: You can't miss this tall drink of water coming down the street! She's pure rock 'n' roll perfection in her signature tangle of tough silver jewelry, always with a cool boot and something made of black leather.

Self-described style: "A mix of a lanky Keith Richards and the Ramones."

Caroline Forsling, designer and model

Why: Because everything she puts on (and I mean *everything*) looks incredible on her.

Self-described style: "My aesthetic is very Swedish— simple, nothing complicated. I love classics, vintage, all things timeless and not trendy: no designer logos or the obvious."

Miguelina Gambaccini, designer

Why: Everyone wants to be the super-feminine and sexy Miguelina, who embodies the glamorous beach lifestyle.

Self-described style: "I think people expect I take all this time to prepare, but I don't! My style is effortless."

Kim Gordon, rock star/artist/writer

Why: Kim has an amazing sense of style that has evolved from vintage/ripped jeans to something more grown-up—yet still as cool as ever. And because, hey, she's Kim Gordon!

Self-described style: "Tomboy lite. I used to wear a lot of band T-shirts."

Molly Guy, founder of Stone Fox Bride

Why: I love how she puts herself together, elevating her Grateful Dead– loving, Indian-hippie pieces with Chanel bags and ballet flats.

Self-described style: "It's pretty easygoing. I don't own many clothes, but the ones I do own, I *love*. I have a few items I return to year after year, like a classic beat-up black leather jacket and vintage Indian cotton block-print dresses. The more ponchos and capes, the better!"

Jamie Haller, creative director, NSF

Why: She has an amazing eye for denim, and she really knows how to style it in a cool and unexpected way.

Self-described style: "Sloppy-sexy, tomboyish and easy, forward and casual."

Susan Houser, makeup artist

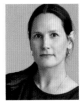

Why: Susan puts herself together in that really chic bohemian way that only she can do.

Self-described style: "Elegant gypsy: a collage of my own vintage mixed with great inexpensive finds and current designer pieces."

April Johnson, stylist and designer, Alasdair

Why: She wears cool items of her own design with pieces by Margiela, Maria Cornejo, and Lauren Manoogian—always with pretty gold jewelry by Ted Muehling. *And* she's an amazing stylist.

Self-described style: "I'm a minimalist, and I love a uniform—comfortable clothes with perfectly tailored details."

Susan Kaufman, consulting fashion editor

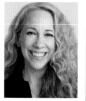

Why: She always looks super put together and classic with a twist. And that amazing hair makes everything look so much cooler!

Self-described style: "Classic chic."

Daryl Kerrigan, fashion designer

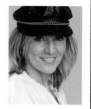

Why: Daryl was the first person to make rock 'n' roll pants that actually fit. And she's the Pied Piper of Cool, as I once described her in *Harper's Bazaar.*

Self-described style: "I love layering, so I've got tons of silk underpinnings, shirts in all fabrics, knits of all types. I have to be able to move freely in my clothes and shoes, so I love sneakers and boots with a walkable heel."

Christina Kornilakis, vintage clothing seller and consultant

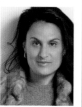

Why: Nobody knows more about vintage and how to wear it than Christina. Plus, she cracks me up.

Self-described style: "Casual sexy."

Tina Lipman, makeup artist

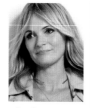

Why: She reminds me of a '70s movie star (think Britt Ekland) and always looks beachy/sexy/cool and casual.

Self-described style: "Feminine, bohemian rocker."

Jeanine Lobell, makeup artist and founder of Stila

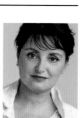

Why: Jeanine is a tough chick who wears what she wants (like a confection of a Chanel dress with espadrilles and punky hair), and it always works.

Self-described style: "Effortless with a bit of an edge."

Pascale Poma, makeup artist

Why: Pascale is just a stunner. Her style is chic and feminine with a touch of humor.

Self-described style: "I like clothes that tell a bit about the way I see the world. I dislike uniformity or prettiness."

Michele Quan, ceramicist

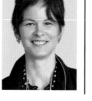

Why: Michele is the epitome of casual cool with a disheveled and comfortable artist style, which she glams up with tons and tons of fine gold and diamond jewelry—many pieces of her own design.

Self-described style: "Girlie tomboy."

Meredith Rollins, editor in chief, *Redbook*

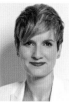

Why: She always looks perfectly European classic.

Self-described style: "Most honestly, 'terrified post-preppy.' If I try something trendy, it's usually from Zara and thus dead cheap. I'm also far more apt to buy clothes that have a cool detail or a fun print but are still classic enough to last for years."

Janis Savitt, jewelry designer

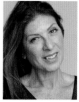

Why: Janis is legendary. She first appeared in one of my all-time favorite books: *Scavullo Women.*

Self-described style: "I would say I'm pretty classic and not the type of person to follow trends; I don't want to look like an uncomfortable fashion victim. Yet I will wear anything from any era—1890 to the present day— and make everything work together."

Karen Schijman, stylist

Why: She is sexy, sexy, sexy in her fierce heels (I have never seen her in flats!), minis, and skinny rocker pants.

Self-described style: "I have always stuck to a version of a uniform. I tend to be attracted to classic men's tailoring with a nod to Yves Saint Laurent 1970s style."

Leigh Shoemaker, stylist and model

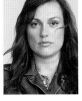

Why: Leigh has a knack for putting together vintage pieces so they look brand-new and chic. And as a full-figure model, she's also an expert on dressing for larger women.

Self-described style: "Classic with an esoteric edge and kind of sexy but always practical."

Gayle Smith, fashion designer

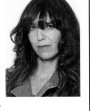

Why: She has the most amazing eye for vintage and for knowing when an iffy piece will look chic with a flick of the wrist—like how she cinches the waist of a military jumpsuit, adds heels, and becomes the most glamorous woman in the room!

Self-described style: "Like most women, I constantly change my style based on my eclectic shopping habits—I'm always looking for something unexpected. While I love minimal, oversize classics, I also go for global, nomadic handcrafted pieces."

Lisa Immordino Vreeland, filmmaker

Why: Lisa looks completely put together but has a slight bohemian edge: the long, uncomplicated hair; her cool everyday Ten Thousand Things pendants on leather; no makeup.

Self-described style: "I am big believer in having a uniform. A blazer with white jeans has been mine for years. I have tried to become a bit more feminine as I've gotten older, and have added dresses to my wardrobe."

Kaela Matranga Wells, art adviser

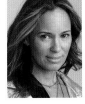

Why: She's got that perfect laid-back California high/low vibe.

Self-described style: "I'm bohemian with an edge, modern European mixed with California ease."

Brooke Williams, lifestyle blogger

Why: I love the way she wears what she's drawn to and then tweaks it to make it all her own. Only Brooke can rock a 1940s suit so it looks 100 percent modern.

Self-described style: "Sentimental. I still wear things I bought in college, that belonged to my grandmother, or that were made by a friend. I've been mixing vintage and modern for as long as I can remember."

Anamaria Wilson, VP of corporate communications, Michael Kors

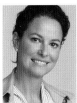

Why: I could only *wish* to look like she does in basic classics!

Self-described style: "Severe chic in winter, boho-chic in summer, and little bit of both in the spring and fall."

Scosha Woolridge, jewelry designer

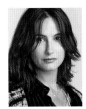

Why: I am obsessed with how she throws herself together in such an easy bohemian way, like she's never really trying. And I love all of her little tattoos.

Self-described style: "Practical, classic, comfortable, bohemian beach tomboy with a vintage feminine edge from the '80s."

WHY DENIM IS EVERYTHING TO ME

You might think it's weird for a style book to start with an entire chapter devoted to denim. Well, I figured, this is *my* style book, and everything jeans-y is what I am all about. I'm most comfortable in a slouchy top, a jacket, and a great pair of skinnies, slight "slouchies," or even bell-bottoms should the mood hit, in blue, black, gray, or white. With heels, the vibe is dressy, while Birkenstocks or clogs convey a running-around-the-city weekend look.

Today you can wear denim pretty much anywhere, but that wasn't always the case. When I worked at *Harper's Bazaar* in the '90s, my boss reprimanded me for wearing jeans to a fashion show. No matter that they were Daryl K and supercute, and that I'd paired them with vintage red wedges and an Agnès B. overcoat for a chic-as-all-get-out ensemble. These days, I only rarely encounter the "no jeans" dress code, usually for a fancy party. Unless you work in a very corporate environment, you can do denim at the office and look perfectly acceptable—while feeling sexy-cool and comfortable in the bargain.

Despite denim's universality, many women still reserve jeans for the weekend. If wearing denim as an everyday staple doesn't come naturally to you, it can be hard to figure out what works, what doesn't, and how to style it. So it makes sense to start with this chapter after all, doesn't it?

The Perfect Pair of Jeans

Jeans are really only cool if they've got everything going for them. This includes the right wash. (Feeling a '70s look? Then go light and wide-leg. Something more chic? Keep it dark, rigid, and straight or authentically faded.) Because I am such a fan, I have every kind of jean under the sun, choosing the pair du jour depending on my mood and what I want to convey on any particular day.

Here, I break down what really good everyday classic five-pocket jeans should look like—because no matter how many other pairs you might have, these are the ones no one should be without.

THE RIGHT WASH ADDS INTEREST. I like a whole range, from super faded to inky-dark. Almost every hue has its place, but skip anything too trendy or tricky like jeans with obvious bleach stains or acid-wash denim—unless you're OK with the fact that their moment will be fleeting.

A LITTLE BIT OF STRETCH GOES A LONG WAY. The right amount of Lycra woven into the fabric makes jeans more comfortable and fit better. Aim for between I and 4 percent; any more can result in unsightly puckers down the back of the thigh, too-shiny denim that looks inauthentic, or just an overall sausage effect.

BACK POCKETS ARE KEY. Their size and siting is crucial! They should be big enough to slimmify your butt: at least four inches across. Tiny pockets or ones placed too high or low can throw off the balance by creating strange proportions or visually enlarging your backside.

THE KNEE CAN DETERMINE WHETHER YOU LOOK LONG-LEGGED OR NOT. Straight-leg jeans should be fitted—not to be confused with tight—along the knee. This will visually lengthen your entire body. Luckily, a too-stovepipe leg is a quick fix at the tailor. Here's how to do it: Face the mirror head-on while wearing your jeans and whatever footwear you'd normally pair them with. Have your tailor pin the sides of the knee area (not all the way down the leg or you'll end up with pegged jodhpurs), carefully blending the new seam back into the existing one. Before making any final alterations, be sure you can easily bend your knees!

Denim for Every Mood

If you're crazy about jeans like I am, you might want to start building your collection now. Here's a sample of what's in my closet.

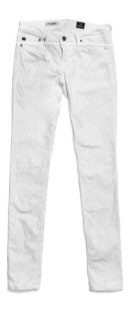

WHITE OR CREAM. Great year-round. Pair with a classic peacoat in the fall, a white tee in the summer.

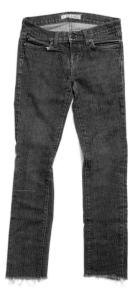

SKINNY BLUE. Dress them up or down—so versatile.

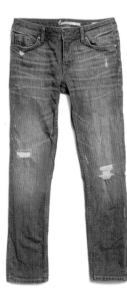

RIPPED AND PATCHED. The key to styling them is contrast: make sure *everything* else on your body is tailored and pristine.

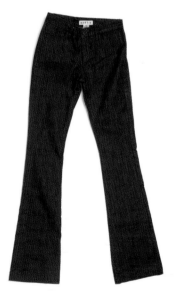
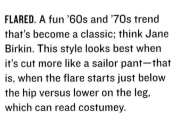

FLARED. A fun '60s and '70s trend that's become a classic; think Jane Birkin. This style looks best when it's cut more like a sailor pant—that is, when the flare starts just below the hip versus lower on the leg, which can read costumey.

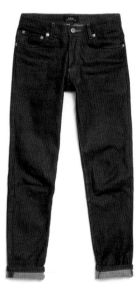

DARK WASH. Surprisingly polished: these look great with a blazer for work.

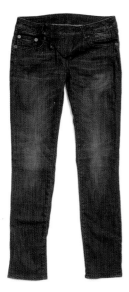

SKINNY BLACK. With the right jewelry and shoes, they can look super dressy.

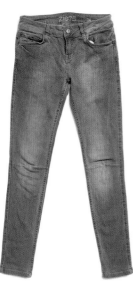

FADED GRAY. Imparts a slightly rock 'n' roll vibe. Looks great with a white, black, or jewel-toned (burgundy, emerald-green) top.

5 Denim Pieces Every Woman Should Own

1. A PAIR OF WORN-IN REGULAR-FIT JEANS THAT YOU FEEL GREAT WEARING—for example, a boyfriend jean that's not too baggy.

2. A GOOD WESTERN-STYLE JACKET WITH LARGE BREAST POCKETS. Small pockets look cheap, fake, and "junior." Search for an authentic vintage version or a well-done reproduction that passes for the real thing.

3. A NICE WIDER-LEG TROUSER-STYLE PANT, either high- or low-waisted (whichever feels right to you).

4. A DARK SKINNY PAIR FOR DRESSING UP (OR DOWN). To preserve the color and prevent fading, dry-clean them or wash inside out in cold water and hang to dry.

5. A DENIM OR CHAMBRAY SHIRT. Any pockets should be at least three inches across so they don't look laughably dinky. (See "A Good Western-Style Jacket," above.)

I Love a Good Denim Jacket

I have been collecting denim jackets for years. You're probably thinking, *Who needs more than one?* Well, most people don't: one really great classic can serve all your needs. But I just love the different washes (faded, ripped, dark) and the many shapes they come in: shrunken for layering, oversize to throw on top of everything, a barn jacket for an old-timey feel.

No matter the style, a good jean jacket should have a few standard characteristics.

My favorite no-name vintage piece

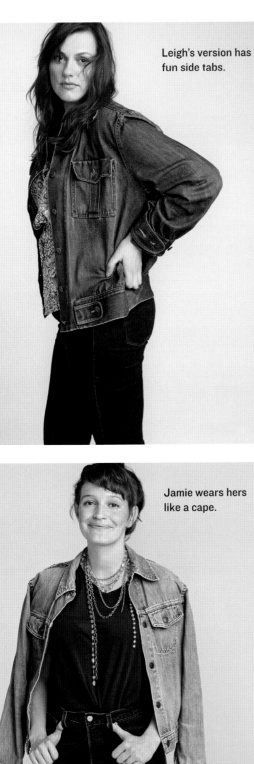

Leigh's version has
fun side tabs.

Brooke's vintage
Lee makes
anything look
cooler.

Jamie wears hers
like a cape.

23

ANATOMY OF

The Perfect Denim Jacket

You can change an outfit dramatically with a great jacket, and that includes my beloved denim versions. But if you don't look for the right characteristics, you won't achieve the cool you're going for. As I've said, I have quite a few versions of my favorite topper—dark, faded, ripped, pristine, and even blazers. But when looking for a great if-you-can-only-have-one piece, go for classic. Here's my stellar vintage Levi's jacket that didn't come 100 percent ideal (I had the slightly blousy '80s arms taken in a tad). Now it's pretty much perfect, and here's why.

A DARK OR SLIGHTLY (AND AUTHENTICALLY) FADED WASH— no trendy splotches.

SLEEVES THAT ARE NARROW ENOUGH TO CREATE A SLEEK SILHOUETTE but wide enough to fit over a sweater.

SLASH POCKETS—always handy!

ADJUSTABLE TABS on the sides of the hem.

A PERFECT-SIZE COLLAR—not too long and pointy, not too short.

TWO BIG BREAST POCKETS. Tiny pockets are too junior-department and cheap-looking.

OLD-SCHOOL METAL BUTTONS, either silver or copper toned.

LEVI STRAUSS & CO.

Denim Goes to the Office

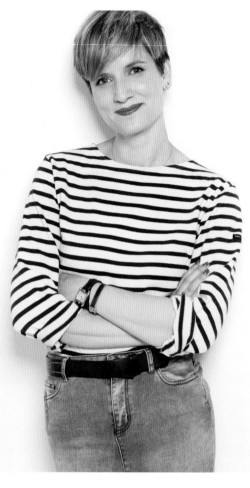

There was a time when it would have been crazy to wear jeans to work (as I learned firsthand at *Harper's Bazaar*). Thankfully, those days are in the past. Of course, if you're a corporate lawyer or a staffer in a very formal office, you may only get away with wearing denim in the workplace on Fridays. That's when to pair dark-wash jeans with a serious silk blouse and tailored jacket, plus high-heeled boots or T-straps. Make sure all shoes, tops, and accessories are classic and/or tailored enough to make the outfit appear polished. But even if your office is pretty lax, don't show up in a too-casual look; save the fun patched jeans for weekends and vacations. In a professional environment, I advise dark-blue, black, gray, or white jeans.

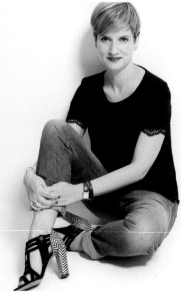

"It's *really* hard for me to wear denim to the office anymore, except on Fridays or days when I don't have corporate meetings. How do I get away with jeans? By wearing heels and a full face of makeup, which somehow distracts from whatever lower-key stuff I've got going on. The striped sailor shirt is a go-to for me; it feels snappy and naval, even though it's a T-shirt. And a black lace top dresses up and feminizes the jeans, while the color says, 'Take me seriously!'"

—Meredith Rollins

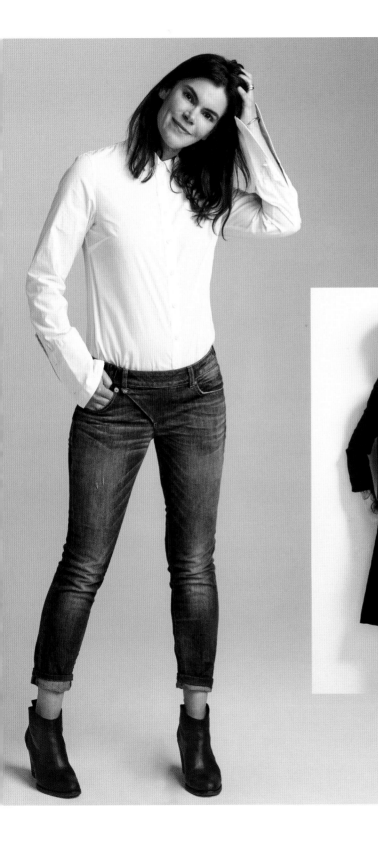

Because she's in a creative field, Anne gets away with jeans for formal meetings by pairing them with a men's slim-cut white shirt, buttoned to the top and tucked in. Leaving her cool French cuffs unbuttoned creates a nice dichotomy. (Equally smart would be the opposite: sleeves done up with cuff links, and the shirt unbuttoned to the sternum so you can see necklaces or just bare skin.) Rounding out Anne's look are rich brown leather ankle boots, which have medium stacked heels and a slightly feminine shape.

Michele is also a creative professional, but when she has to meet with serious people, she simply throws together a jacket (like this cool Rachel Comey duster) and a vintage satin vest to go with her jeans.

CHEAT SHEET

Office Denim

Denim can look professional, as long as you keep everything else spare and elegant. Here are some options.

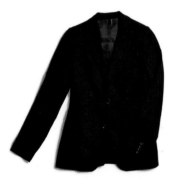

A BEAUTIFULLY TAILORED BLAZER. A menswear suit jacket with two or three buttons (or double-breasted) that fits well in the shoulders will look fresh for years. The most classic look is for the jacket to hit right at the middle of your butt. A feminine collarless, buttonless jacket works as a nice alternative.

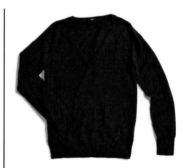

A BLACK OR DARK-BLUE HIGH-QUALITY FITTED CREW- OR V-NECK CASHMERE SWEATER. Better quality equals less chance of pilling, which looks unkempt. (You don't have to spend a fortune: J. Crew uses good cashmere and makes great silhouettes.)

PUMPS IN LEATHER OR SUEDE. Try a pointy-toed pair to convey fierce sexiness, or a round toe for a more classic, feminine look.

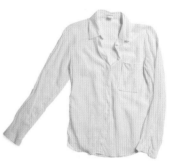

A SOLID CREAM OR BLACK DRAPEY SILK BUTTON-DOWN, SHELL, OR TIE-NECK BLOUSE. Neutral shades strike a more serious note.

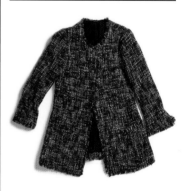

A CHANEL-STYLE BOUCLÉ JACKET. This will upgrade any pair of jeans to chic French-girl status.

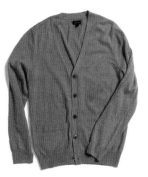

A MAN'S OVERSIZE CASHMERE CARDIGAN. Try it buttoned up over just a silk camisole and add big earrings for a party, or wear it over a blouse or crisp shirt at work.

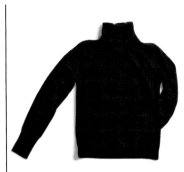

A BODY-SKIMMING (READ: NOT TIGHT) THIN-KNIT TURTLENECK. Go for black, navy, camel, or dark heather gray in rich merino wool or cashmere.

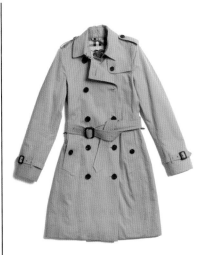

A TRENCH COAT. Always timeless—and it makes a pair of jeans (even patched ones) look tony.

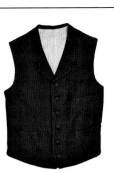

A MEN'S-STYLE CLASSIC SUIT VEST. This piece adds a fun element, whether worn under a cardigan or blazer or over a white tee.

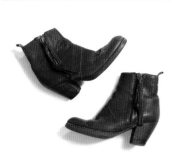

CLASSIC ANKLE BOOTS. They should be relatively fitted in the ankle (a wide ankle looks cheap and ruins most silhouettes), and feature a mid to high heel that's relatively narrow.

TIP: You can also slip denim pieces into your regular work looks. Try a chambray or thin denim shirt with a skirt suit, or swap your wool blazer for a dark denim one instead.

Jeans Are Perfect for Parties

Unless the invite says "no jeans," they are the best pants for any festivity. Why? Because jeans are comfortable and chic and a blank canvas for any cocktail look. Heed the office rule: choose a dark wash and leave the ripped pairs at home.

My favorite jeans are party-worthy when I throw on my metallic Gregory Parkinson wrap kimono and Terry De Havilland wedges. No one can say I'm "just wearing jeans"!

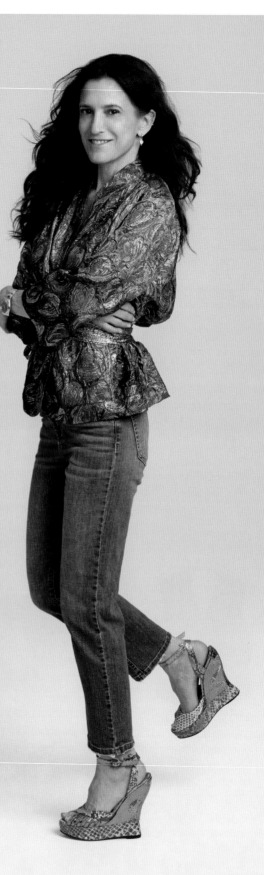

Turn Jeans into a Party Outfit with These Additions

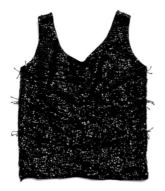

A PARTY TOP. Think feminine shapes or modern "statement" tops like tunics or shells. Also, festive pieces with either exaggerated puffed sleeves or more straightforward cuts—in satin, lace, chiffon, sequins, and unwashed silk.

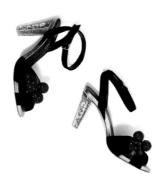

FUN SANDALS OR SEXY HIGH-HEELED PUMPS. Red, beaded, or metallic equals festive. Also good: pointy-toed T-straps, Mary Janes, sling backs, and d'Orsay pumps.

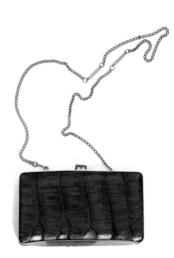

A CHIC LITTLE EVENING BAG. A clutch or a long-chain-strapped purse (in leather, satin, or suede) is a good option.

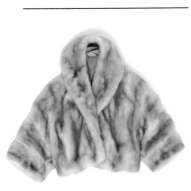

A FAUX-FUR JACKET. Always a fun accent piece.

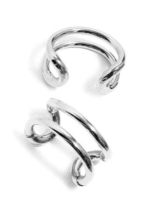

BOLD JEWELRY. Cuffs, chandelier earrings, diamonds—pick one piece and let it be the star.

TIP: Wear stronger makeup than usual. Smoky eyes or red lips are all you need.

Delving into Denim with Jennifer Alfano, Fashion Writer and Jewelry Designer

What are your favorite jeans?

My Current/Elliott boyfriend jeans get the most play, followed by a J. Brand skinny pair—which has the perfect fit. I also love wide-leg ones, including an old pair of J. Brands that are great with a fitted shirt and clogs or heels.

Describe your go-to denim outfit.

Boyfriend jeans, a button-down shirt (silk Madewell or Equipment if I'm dressing up, cotton if I'm going casual), a blazer (Phillip Lim or an old Balenciaga), and either sneakers or wedges from Céline, depending on whether I'm running around or dressing up. And layers of necklaces, always.

How do you dress up jeans?

With a printed silk blouse (A.L.C. or Derek Lam) and my classic Manolo Blahnik black suede BB pumps. Sometimes, I'll cover up with a blazer or my Nili Lotan black leather moto jacket.

What accessories are key to your denim look?

My jewelry. Every piece of jewelry I design, especially my pendants, is something to be worn every day—which in my case means with jeans. If it can't work with jeans, I don't make it! I also like Isabel Marant belts, which are a necessity with boyfriend styles. I often wear black jeans in the winter, paired with a blue denim button-down. I have an ancient child-size Wrangler jacket that I wear in the summer with sundresses. And I love a knee-length classic denim skirt in the warmer months with heels and a blouse . . . superchic.

Jennifer rarely dresses down, so even in jeans she always looks very upper-crust and polished. Key is her choice of jackets and shoes. Here, she pairs denim with a soft French-style jacket and streamlined heels.

City Jeans, Country Jeans

Laura wears jeans all the time, whether she's running around the city, styling on set, or laboring in her other role as an upstate farmer (she owns Westwind Orchard with her husband, fashion photographer Fabio Chizzola). In Manhattan, she pairs them with sleek ankle boots, a short navy peacoat, and a structured designer tote. At the farm, Laura goes for a pair of baggy overalls, a diaphanous Indian hippie top, and Hunter boots.

"Jeans are all you need—they are versatile, chic, functional, sexy, and comfortable. City and country are almost interchangeable to me: I love wearing Birkenstocks with any jeans—from my vintage Levi's to high-waist Wranglers, which work well for either location. Sometimes, I'll dress up denim with a heel and a menswear jacket. Statement jewelry looks great and not precious."

—Laura Ferrara

10 Great Pieces for Styling Jeans in the City

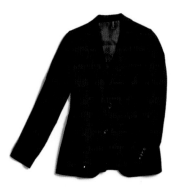

1. A CLASSIC BLAZER. Navy, black, or camel; tweed or plaids (subtle houndstooth or glen plaid); and brushed white or khaki cotton (so crisp in summer!) are nice options.

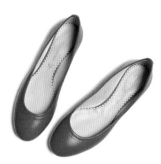

2. BALLET FLATS OR MID- OR HIGH-HEELED ANKLE BOOTS

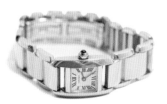

3. A STRUCTURED LEATHER TOTE in black, tan, brown, navy, or red

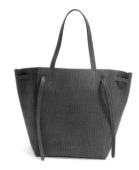

4. A GOOD WATCH like a classic Cartier tank (or similar) with a leather or lizard band. Or a chunky men's-style timepiece with a stainless-steel bracelet.

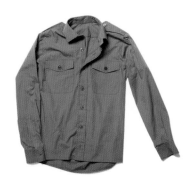

5. A TUCKED-IN REGULATION ARMY SHIRT (very French) or denim or cotton-poplin shirt under an easy cashmere sweater

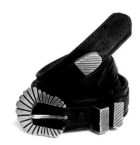

6. A STATEMENT BELT somehow makes jeans feel complete.

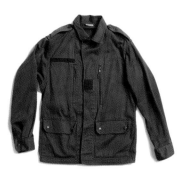

7. A FRENCH OR ITALIAN ARMY JACKET or a longer lightweight duster jacket

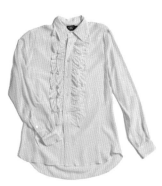

9. A PLEATED OR RUFFLE-FRONT TUXEDO SHIRT (French cuffs? Even better!)

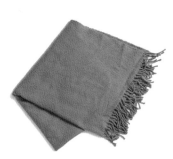

8. A LARGE SCARF. I like a cashmere one in winter—ideally black, camel, gray, or plaid. And Matta's cotton *dupattas* are perfect for spring through fall.

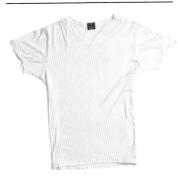

10. A SIMPLE WHITE OR BLACK COTTON V- OR CREW-NECK TEE is the ideal blank canvas—it can be worn in myriad ways, whether on its own or layered.

All Hail the Canadian Tuxedo

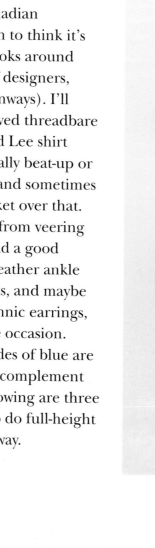

Me in my favorite classic denim "suit"

Here's one of my all-time favorite looks: the double-denim "suit." Although many people shun denim-on-denim—otherwise known as the Canadian tuxedo—I happen to think it's one of the best looks around (and so do lots of designers, judging by the runways). I'll half-tuck my beloved threadbare and multi-patched Lee shirt into a pair of equally beat-up or very dark jeans—and sometimes layer a denim jacket over that. To keep the look from veering too "trucker," I add a good pair of mid-heel leather ankle boots or sexy heels, and maybe some dangling ethnic earrings, depending on the occasion. Although the shades of blue are all different, they complement one another. Following are three other women who do full-height denim their own way.

"I've always loved the color of denim. This outfit is a no-brainer to put on, and so flattering. It's like a blank canvas. I always love a good menswear shirt, and the shape of these pants looks really good on women: high-waist pants elongate your body."

—Maria Cornejo

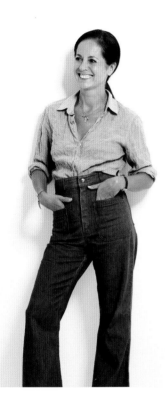 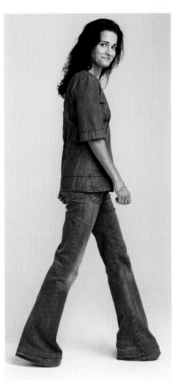 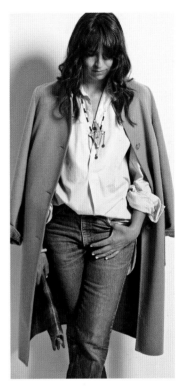

The Look: Euro-boyish

Maria pairs a men's soft chambray shirt (of her own design) with a pair of vintage high-waist regulation sailor jeans.

WHY IT WORKS: The two shades meld together to create the effect of a jumpsuit, and the exaggerated higher waist makes for an elegant look that doesn't say "ranch hand."

The Look: Feminine Cool

Anna wears a short-sleeved tunic made of lightweight denim over a pair of super-wide-leg jeans.

WHY IT WORKS: The flare's effect is that of an elegant long dress, which lengthens her body.

The Look: Urban Chic

Gayle breaks up head-to-toe denim by throwing a camel-colored coat over boyfriend jeans and a super-faded chambray shirt, and adding a vintage beaded Maasai necklace.

WHY IT WORKS: You can't get more classic than a camel coat: it's the perfect complement to faded or dark denim, immediately dressing it up.

Mixing Denims

Now that we've eased into and embraced the whole denim-on-denim thing, it's time to branch out and try different shades together. I love pairing black and blue, whether it's a chambray shirt and dark, inky jeans or the other way around—a faded black denim shirt looks great with faded or super-dark blue jeans, and even gray ones. White jeans always work with dark or beat-up denim shirts and jackets, and I also have a good white denim shirt that I wear with blue or black jeans. In other words, it's all good.

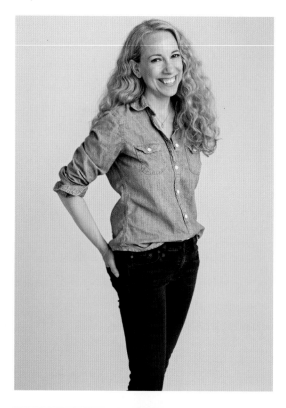

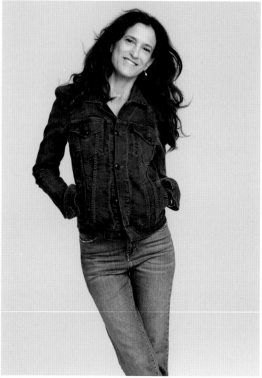

BLACK DENIM (ON BLUE DENIM): Even though Susan and I are wearing different denim shades, the outfits work in both cases: my black jacket looks sleek with the blue jeans, and Susan's classic chambray shirt is elevated when she pairs it with skinny black jeans.

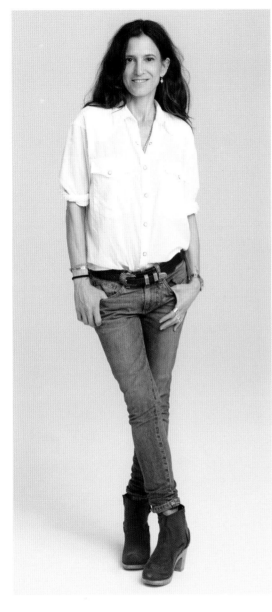

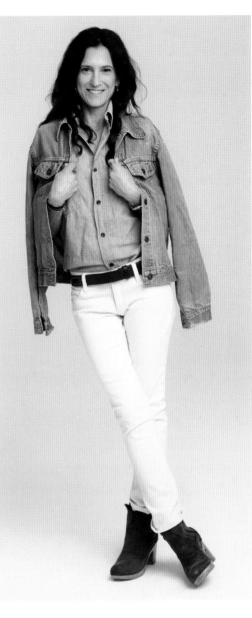

My white Western-style denim shirt with blue jeans is a more casual way to rock the white button-down.

And the opposite works too!

TIP: When donning head-to-toe denim, keep accessories to a minimum—a chunky watch or big hoop earrings are all you need.

Wear Ripped Jeans and Look Perfectly Acceptable

Slightly torn jeans have become a wardrobe staple; seemingly every designer has made his or her own version. To up the chic factor, pair them with fancier pieces, like Kaela does here, keeping the rest of your outfit—including shoes and bags—neat and sharp. Her structured white blazer and twisted evening top dress up the jeans, while the straw menswear hat and platform espadrilles lend the right amount of funk. (Hanging around the house watching old movies is the only time to wear them with other ripped pieces, like your favorite old Grateful Dead tee.)

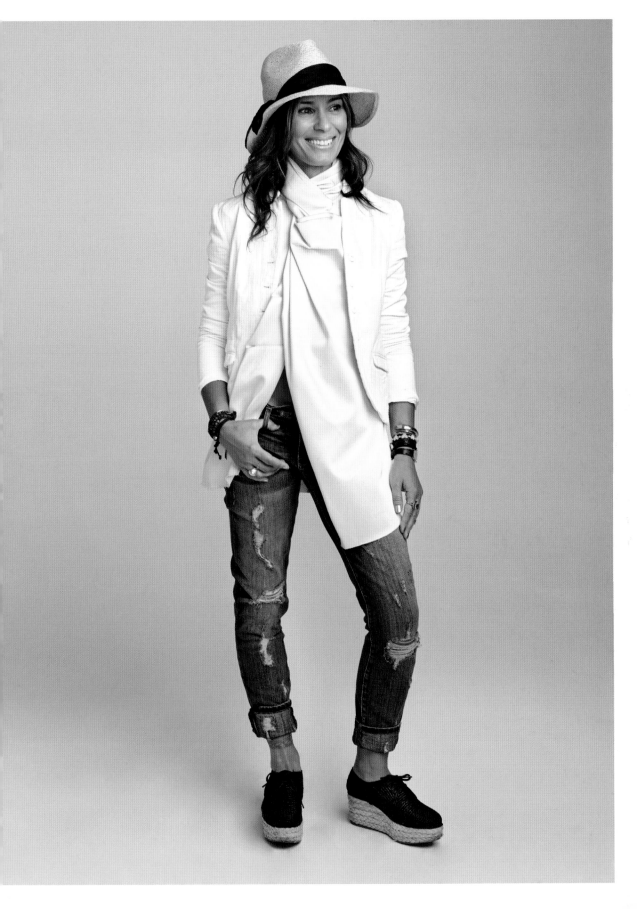

What Works with Ripped Jeans

Let the jeans be the one crazy piece. Here are some classic, sensible options to go with your favorite beat-up pair.

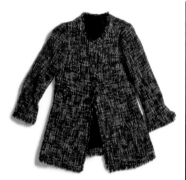

A STRUCTURED BLAZER IN TWEED OR TROPICAL WOOL. Try a classic navy one with gold buttons, or an English schoolboy style.

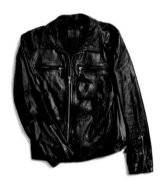

A BUTTERY-SOFT LEATHER JACKET WITH SIMPLE LINES. Go with a blazer, zip-front, or peacoat style. (A full-on biker jacket would be too much.)

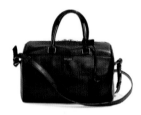

A GOOD LEATHER BAG. A top-handle satchel is posh enough to elevate the jeans a few notches.

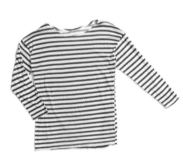

A FRENCH STRIPED BOAT TOP. Wear one of these for a sweet and gamine look.

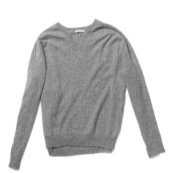

RICH-LOOKING CASHMERE SWEATERS. V-necks, crew necks, and men's-style cardigans in shades like camel, navy, and black are the most appropriate.

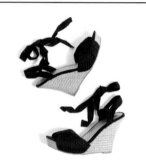

CHIC WEDGES. Espadrilles are great for summer, wooden-heeled ones in fall.

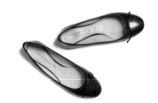

BLACK (OR RED) BALLET FLATS. For a perfect French touch.

For More Ripped-Jean Outfits, Just Add . . .

FALL

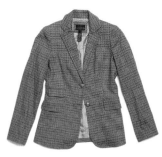

• A TWEED JACKET

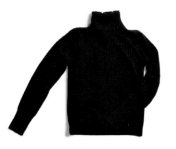

• A THIN TURTLENECK

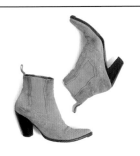

• ANKLE BOOTS

SPRING

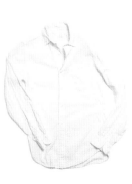

• A CRISP WHITE MEN'S SHIRT
  (NOT TOO BAGGY!)

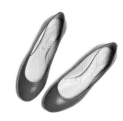

• RED OR BLACK BALLET FLATS

PARTY

• BIG ETHNIC EARRINGS

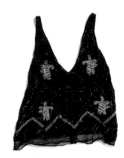

• A SEQUINED TOP

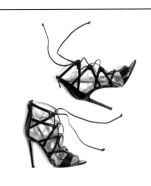

• STRAPPY HEELS

5 Ways to Personalize Your Jeans

1. **FIX ANY HOLES FROM UNDERNEATH** at the tailor for a cool patchwork effect.

2. **FOLD THEM INTO A SUPERWIDE CUFF** at the bottom to create cool drama.

3. **HACK OFF THE HEMS** for a casual frayed effect (this looks great when paired with fancy shoes). Once you wash the jeans, the hems will start to fray naturally.

4. **CHANGE YOUR BELT** to change your look: a gold sequined or jeweled piece for a slightly dressy vibe, a leather cowboy one—complete with silver buckle—for a cool western feel.

5. **MAKE PERFECT BEACH CUTOFFS.** Snip them at a slight angle: lower at the outer thigh than the crotch. This creates a more flattering shape on the leg.

TAILORING TIP: I accidentally splattered red dye on my favorite white jeans, and instead of ditching them, I cut little holes around the stains and had the tailor under-patch them with white denim. The result: a one-of-a-kind pair for weekend wear. (Patches can be good, but stains never are!)

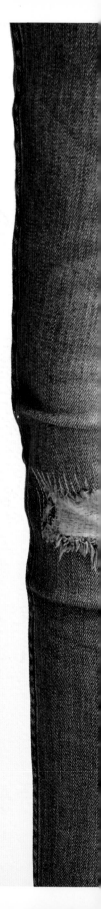

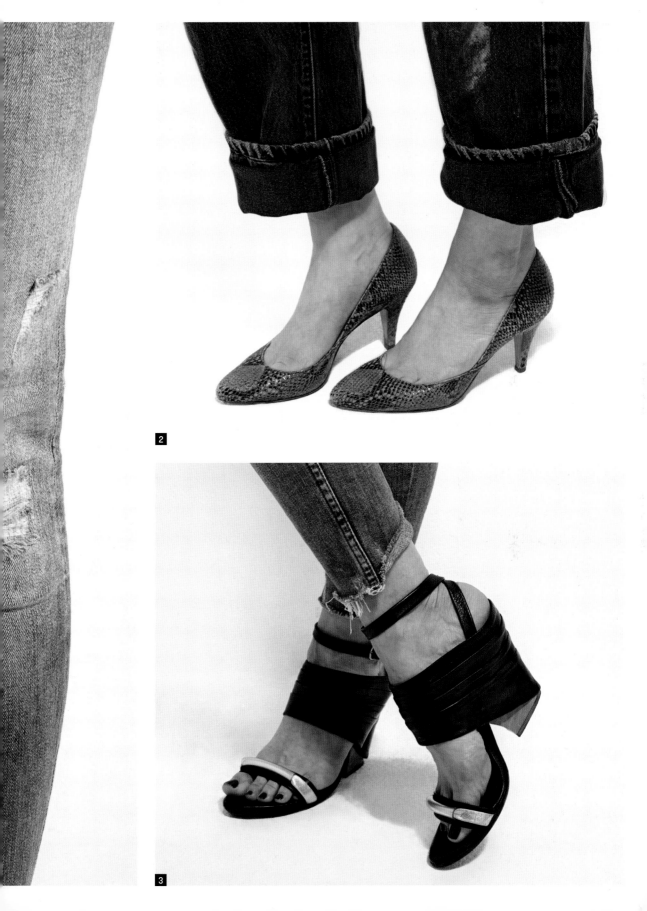

2

3

Getting the Most Out of Your Wardrobe

Embrace Seasonless Dressing

Having separate "summer" and "winter" closets is a rather old-fashioned concept (aside from storing bathing suits and shorts away to make room for sweaters, of course). When I was working at *Lucky* magazine, one of my favorite features to produce was "Now & Later," where we would show how to wear a summer piece in February—because that's when that warm-weather stuff hits stores. Note that it's easier to wear summer pieces in the winter than the other way around. Although on a non-humid summer day, I've been known to rock my Anna (annanyc.com) leather wrap skirt with No.6 clogs and a tee.

Anne has always worn summery cotton kurta tops (available at Do Kham in New York City) year-round, and so have I. Many women reserve them for warmer seasons, but they look especially good with heavier wool and cashmere pieces. I love Anne's blue version with her black pants and coat. And the way she carries a giant French straw market bag as an everyday tote is beyond chic!

FOR A PERFECT FALL LOOK, Anne mixes her simple coat, pants, and ankle boots with a summery top and bag.

You can winterize just about anything like Leigh
cleverly does with her vintage summer dress.

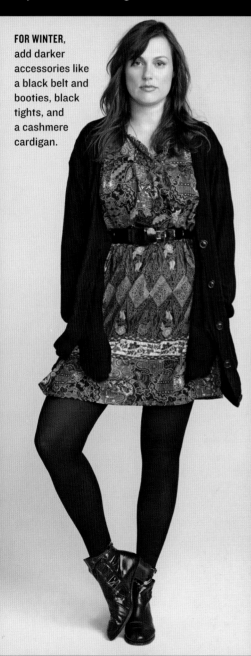

FOR WINTER,
add darker
accessories like
a black belt and
booties, black
tights, and
a cashmere
cardigan.

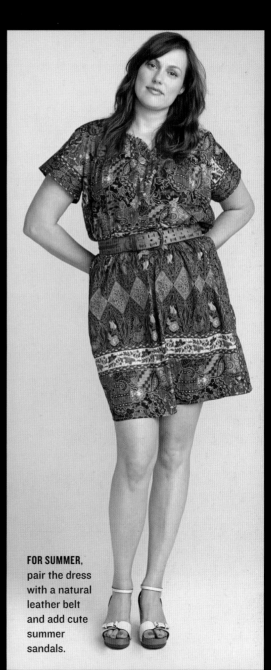

FOR SUMMER,
pair the dress
with a natural
leather belt
and add cute
summer
sandals.

Q&A with Laura Ferrara, Stylist and Farmer

Who are your style icons?

Diane Keaton, Lauren Hutton, Monica Vitti, Françoise Hardy, and Jane Birkin. They dress with such great confidence and ease—it's understated but definitive.

Describe your beauty routine, including products used.

Living Proof No Frizz Nourishing Styling Cream, natural organic beeswax lip balm, Captain Blankenship Organic Sunshine Body Cream, Brooklyn Herborium Nourish and Replenish Oil, Radice Illuminating Mask.

What are the items in your closet that you've had the longest and will never throw out?

Sixteen-year-old broken-in Levi's, original worn-in Helmut Lang jeans, Stan Smiths (that I've had for ages), a Lee denim jacket from the '70s, washed out from wear.

Name some fashion rules you live by.

Comfort—on the farm and on set, comfort is premium. That doesn't necessarily mean sweatpants and a T-shirt, but I'm also not going to style a photo shoot in platform boots, or farm in leather overalls.

Less is more—simple, well-made pieces like a crisp white shirt or tailored trousers and Adidas will speak volumes over layered trendy jewelry.

Quality over quantity—as a stylist, I'm constantly surrounded by clothes, so I try to keep my personal wardrobe staples to a minimum. It takes me a while to commit to a purchase, because I want to make sure I'll really use it for years to come, whether it be my giant black leather Céline tote or my vintage military jacket.

Practicality—on any given day, I'll be in meetings with photographers, and consulting on shoots, while at the same time coordinating farm events and hand delivering eggs for Westwind Orchard. These require functional, practical pieces, and I always keep that in mind when dressing.

Have your own look—just because it's trendy, that doesn't necessarily mean you should buy it.

What did you used to wear all the time that you wouldn't dream of wearing now?

Shorts.

Is there anything you do that breaks conventional fashion rules?

I suppose it's become fashionable again, but I've always shopped from the men's section for pants, T-shirts, and button-downs. The slim fits drape quite nicely (not to mention comfortably) on the female form. It's that simple, understated ease. I'll also shop at army/navy surplus stores and *real* outdoor/work wear stores (e.g., Carhartt, Woolrich, Filson) for jumpsuits, jackets, and pants.

Any good styling tricks? Belting, layering, rolling, cropping?

You can make a belt out of anything (rope, a men's tie, metal chains, strips of leather). And you can affix it in infinite ways, like tied in a sailor's knot, a woven knot, or a giant knot (even if it has a buckle) or fastened with a pin, a big brooch, or even an earring.

Cuffs on tops and bottoms are always flattering to highlight the wrists/forearms and ankles. When it comes to trousers, tailor your pants if possible (it's not necessarily expensive and makes all the difference).

Play with proportions. It's an easy way to update old looks—in the summer wear a long skirt with a flat sandal, and in the winter switch that out for a heavy pair of tights and a tall boot.

Do you have any fashion pet peeves?

Buying something just because it's "on trend." I recently read the quote "Only dead fish follow the stream." The dead fish are my biggest pet peeve.

Do you have any family beauty secrets that have been passed down or have stuck with you?

My grandmother used to grow chamomile on our farm in Italy and in the summers she'd mix it with lemon and spray it in my hair while I lay out in the sun. (My hair used to be very blond.) She also passed down using dried polenta as an exfoliating face wash, and organic olive oil for moisturizing, which I still do today.

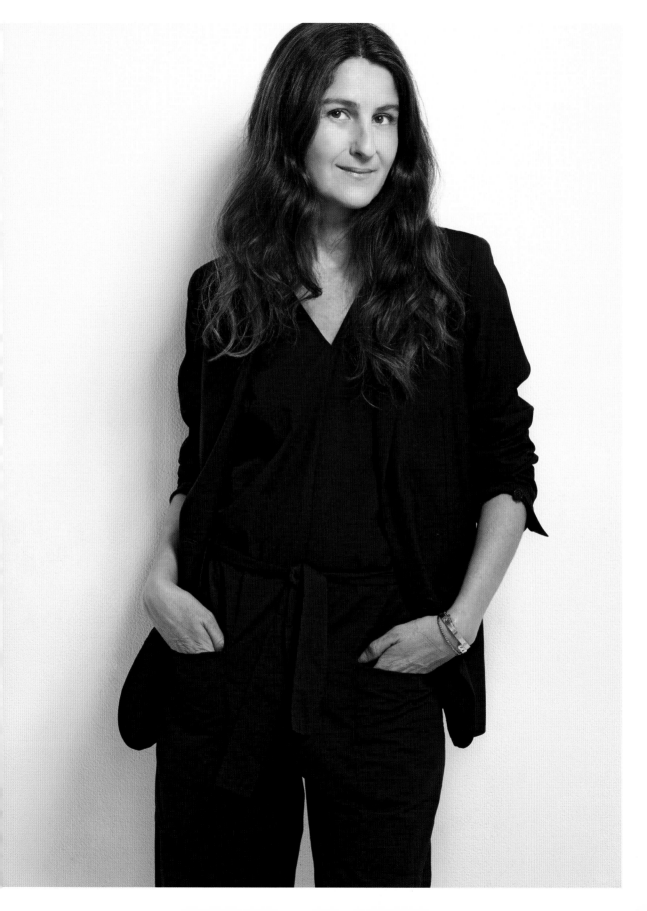

CLASSICS ARE THE BACKBONE OF EVERY CLOSET

Clothes with everlasting style should be the basis of any good wardrobe. But if you don't have the right references, the word *classic* might only conjure up images of wide-wale corduroy or twinsets and a strand of pearls. Classics, instead, are things that have a timeless cut; are made from long-lasting, high-quality fabrics; and mix and match well with a variety of other pieces. And you might just be surprised at what these pieces are.

For instance, I will never throw out my favorite black leather biker jacket. Ever. Or my ankle-high cowboy boots or my mom's amazing hand-sewn brown leather saddlebag from the '70s. Just because these things are each a little bit rock 'n' roll or edgy doesn't mean they are any less classic. On the flip side, well-made "preppier" pieces should be considered for their high quality and ability to stand the test of time. A great-fitting pair of simple trousers and a really high-grade cashmere sweater should also be part of your classic wardrobe—they make anything else you're wearing look that much richer.

The key to keeping classics from looking too boring is to mix them with pieces that have a stronger personality. Sometimes, a plain navy wool blazer is exactly what you need when you're wearing leather pants. The power of classics is all in the way you rock them.

What Makes a Classic?

Why didn't the men of the '80s look as specifically "eighties" as the women? Because menswear cuts usually adhere to a few standard and simple lines. For example, men's shirts have just a few collars to choose from, and those collars have been the same for years. On the other hand, women's tops over the decades have had not only myriad collar styles but also lots of different shapes, lengths, and additions; you could probably spot a ladies' sweater from 1983 a mile away courtesy of its exaggerated shoulders and dolman sleeves.

The takeaway is that if you're on the hunt for classics, you should look for clothes that are cut and tailored simply. Avoid trendy, exaggerated shapes like giant shoulders, very long or cropped lengths, and anything other than a regulation menswear or mandarin collar on a button-down shirt. Think about vintage menswear from your grandfather's day—it still looks totally fresh.

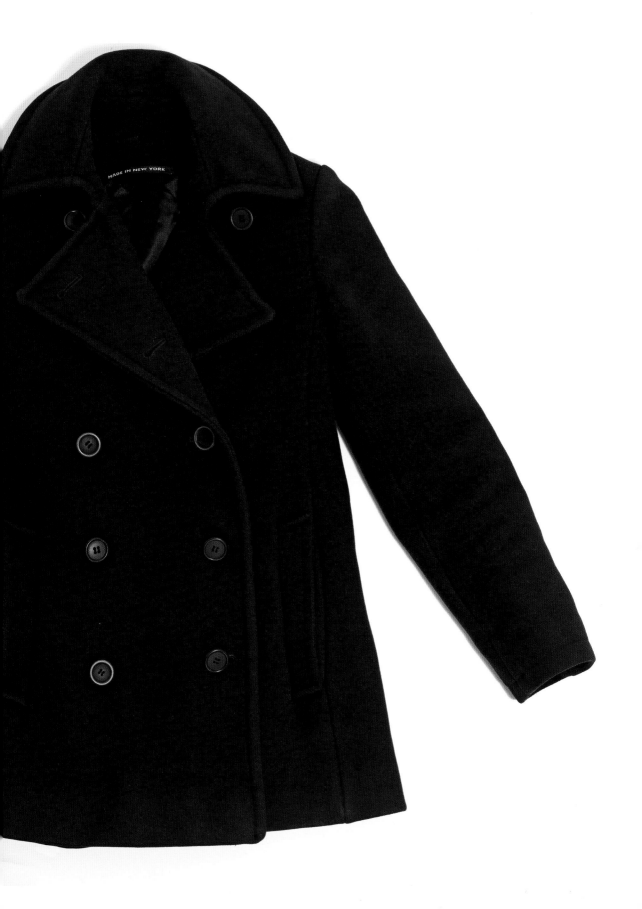

CHEAT SHEET

Classic All-Stars

Check these off your list, and your wardrobe options will be infinite. All are neutral enough to work with any style, and with any other pieces in your arsenal.

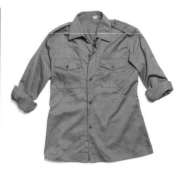

FRENCH ARMY SHIRTS. One of these can replace just about any top in any situation, and can even be worn with an evening skirt and big, dangly earrings.

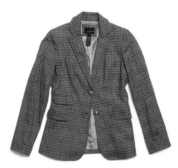

TWO- OR THREE-BUTTON BLAZERS. These are well suited to every occasion, not just the office. Wear them over tees, fancier blouses, cardigans, denim jackets, and even flowy dresses.

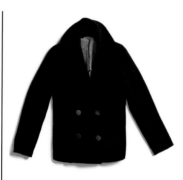

DOUBLE-BREASTED PEACOATS. Think Ali McGraw in *Love Story*—pure perfection.

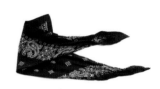

BLUE, BLACK, OR RED BANDANAS. These colorful hankies look cute twisted around your neck, or tied on your head at the beach.

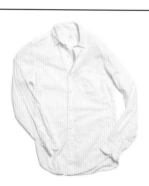

WHITE BUTTON-DOWNS. There are literally thousands of ways to wear a white button-down. This is the blank canvas of your wardrobe.

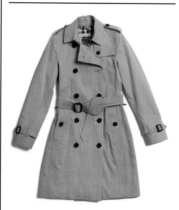

TRENCH COATS. Any outfit you slip one over becomes more serious and a bit more French. A trench works with any style; even punk rockers wear them (albeit to achieve a slightly weird, old English-y vibe).

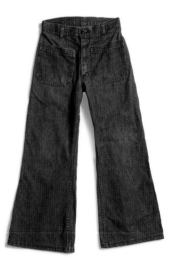

SAILOR SHIRTS/PANTS. A nautical touch is fresh in spring and summer.

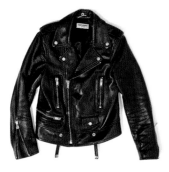

BIKER JACKETS. Keep everything else polished to avoid the mutton-dressed-as-lamb scenario.

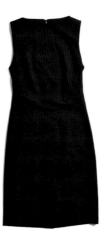

SHIFT DRESSES. Go for one in tropical wool. You can pair it with sandals or more office-appropriate footwear. Feel free to throw a blazer or cardigan over it, too.

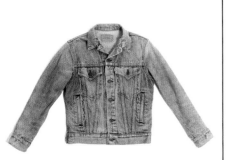

DENIM JACKETS. You can wear a classic Levi's jacket until you're eighty and beyond.

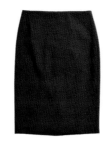

WOOL OR DENIM PENCIL SKIRTS. These versatile pieces transform easily from daytime to nighttime with a simple change of shoes.

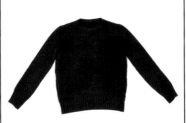

CASHMERE SWEATERS. Superchic and supersoft, these layering pieces amplify the richness and comfort of any outfit.

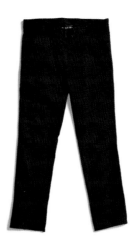

MENSWEAR TROUSERS. I love them a little slouchy—slouchy being the whole point of menswear on women!—and paired with a skimpy tee and a shrunken jacket.

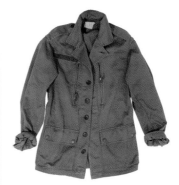

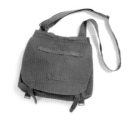

ARMY/NAVY JACKETS, PANTS, SHIRTS, AND BAGS. I love mixing regulation military pieces with more tailored ones. For example, an olive-drab button-down or jacket—my favorite is the French army version shown—worn with a pencil skirt and heels. So Parisian!

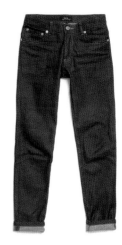

STRAIGHT-LEG JEANS. These will never become outdated, and they can be worn pretty much anywhere. Dark indigo and naturally faded are the best choices.

Classic Fabrics

Clothes made in these materials are always worth a second look: they're timeless, they wear well, and they symbolize quality. If the piece is cut right, go for it.

CASHMERE. The ultimate fabric for knitwear. Stays soft, looks rich, and keeps its shape. It's great for scarves, cardigans, pullovers—anything sweaterlike!

KHAKI. The ultimate spring and fall fabric for classic chinos—which look great rolled up with a strappy heel and a blazer or trench.

DENIM. This fabric speaks for itself. Keep it dark (indigo, black, gray) or naturally faded (even with rips and holes).

SILK. Blouses and camisoles made of silk give any outfit a sense of sophistication and look especially great with wool pieces and jeans.

WOOL. Heavy, tropical-weight, pinstriped, and glen plaid are all fair game. Wool skirts, jackets, trousers, and dresses work in so many situations—especially those where you need to be a bit polished.

OXFORD CLOTH. This is the ultimate preppy fabric. I especially like Polo Ralph Lauren oxford button-downs. (Don't forget to unbutton the collar buttons.)

TWEED. Imparts an upper-crust British vibe and perfectly offsets tough pieces like leather pants.

CORDUROY. I love a good pinwale five-pocket jean or a medium-wale blazer. Corduroy is collegiate in the most charming way.

PLAID FLANNEL. This was a classic way before grunge hit the scene. Wear plaid flannel shirts loose and half-tucked with skinny jeans, or fitted with baggy or high-waisted trousers.

CHAMBRAY. I love a chambray shirt to dress down darker denim jeans, wool pants, or a skirt.

VELVET. Blazers in black, deep blue, or burgundy velvet make an ensemble dressier and a bit stage-worthy.

COTTON SHIRTING. For button-downs, I prefer it really soft and thin.

BOUCLÉ. Pieces made with this fabric look very Chanel and ladylike.

MOLESKIN. This is one of my favorite fabrics for coats and jackets, for its softness and ease.

My Favorite Classic Brands

When shopping for great pieces, start with these trusted brands.

L.L. BEAN. Great for foul-weather necessities, winter jackets, footwear, slippers, and flannel bathrobes.

J. CREW. The best for everything! Cashmere sweaters, tees, coats, trousers, and leather accessories.

FILSON. Amazing hunting jackets— I like them to be a bit oversize.

CHURCH'S SHOES. This English label makes perfect classic Jodhpur boots and lace-up oxfords.

FERRAGAMO. The mid-heel and high-heeled bow pumps can be worn seriously or ironically with punkier pieces like biker jackets and ripped jeans.

LOUIS VUITTON. I'm a sucker for a classic monogram Speedy (the best sizes are 30, 35, and 40— anything smaller is too twee).

RALPH LAUREN. Go here for boys' Polo oxfords and pieces from RRL, which has a great vintage cowboy vibe.

BURBERRY. The best trench coats ever.

THEORY. Season after season, this label never disappoints with its sleek trousers, polished dresses, and great jackets. Head here to build a work wardrobe at a great price.

LEVI'S. There's nothing cooler than these jeans or one of their denim jackets—pieces you will truly have for a lifetime.

A.P.C. Classic French perfection.

MANOLO BLAHNIK. For pumps and evening shoes. They're expensive but will never, ever look dated.

FRYE. No one makes a better harness boot. (Just be wary of their "trend" pieces, which tend to read young.)

NO.6. The best clogs and clog boots in existence—and their silhouettes have more sex appeal than the basic Swedish ones.

UNIQLO. Go here for chic yet inexpensive outerwear, affordable cashmere sweaters, menswear, and great designer collaborations.

Keep Things Interesting by Mixing It Up

I like to see all classics mixing and mingling, and that includes leather pants and suede jackets getting together with tried-and-true fabrics like wool and corduroy. The key to great personal style is knowing how to pair a timeless piece you've had for decades with something of the edgy classic variety.

Try wearing a leather or suede jacket with more serious pieces like a good pair of light wool trousers or a pencil skirt, thereby giving them a little edge. Choose one with a classic cut—not too big or small—and without too many embellishments, although a good vintage fringe suede jacket works well with jeans.

Jennifer makes a cool suede safari jacket look even more timeless by pairing it with her go-to black trousers. Wearing the jacket closed strikes a more serious note, while simply unbuttoning it and letting the belt hang would make it more casual.

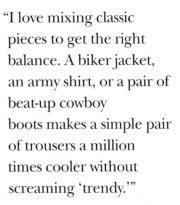

"I love mixing classic pieces to get the right balance. A biker jacket, an army shirt, or a pair of beat-up cowboy boots makes a simple pair of trousers a million times cooler without screaming 'trendy.'"

—Jennifer Alfano

CHEAT SHEET

Fresh Combos

These unexpected pairings keep classics from ever feeling suburban or staid.

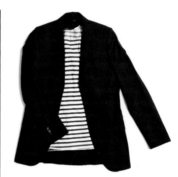

Thin **FRENCH SAILOR'S SHIRT** under a **SUIT** (instead of the expected shell or blouse)

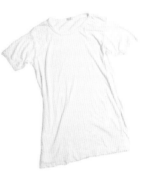

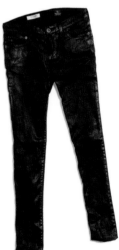

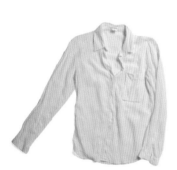

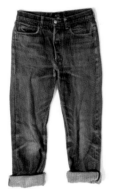

Black or cream **SILK BOW BLOUSE** with **BEAT-UP JEANS**

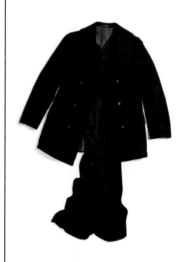

PEACOAT over a **GOWN** (looks so much more interesting than a fancy coat!)

MEN'S WHITE TEE with **SKINNY LEATHER PANTS** and loafers

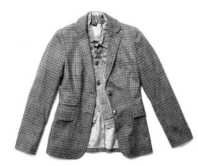

Shrunken **DENIM JACKET** under a **TWEED BLAZER**

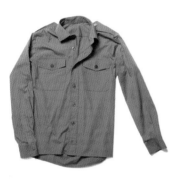

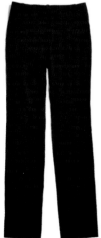

ARMY SHIRT tucked into classic **WOOL TROUSERS**

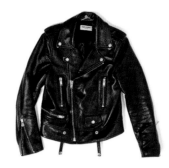

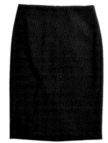

BIKER JACKET and **PENCIL SKIRT**

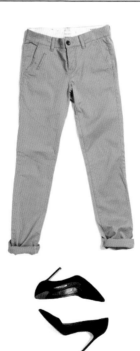

Slightly **BAGGY CHINOS**—rolled up just so—paired with black **POINTY-TOED PUMPS**

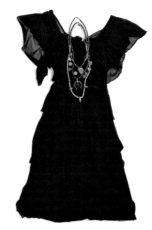

Black **EVENING DRESS** with bold silver **NATIVE AMERICAN JEWELRY**

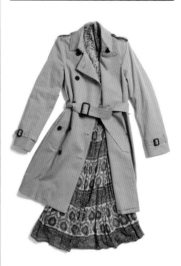

TRENCH COAT over a **HIPPIE DRESS**

Classic Outerwear You'll Wear Forever

I'm all about a great jacket or coat since it's the piece that completes an outfit and can take it from so-so to spectacular. If you're wearing something simple, what you throw over it helps define whatever look you're going for. A giant parka says, "I'm just being easy, casual, and warm" while a good trench gives instant French status with an air of mystery.

A WARM PARKA. Aside from being completely practical, there's something chic about a slightly oversize winter jacket (and it actually makes your legs look thinner!).

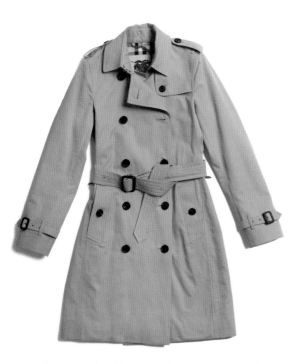

A TRENCH. The ultimate gamine piece, it can swing serious or playful.

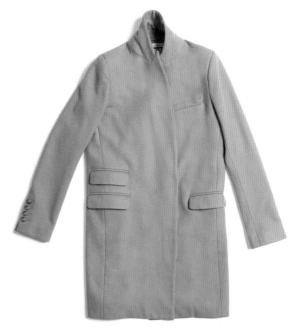

A SHORTER PEACOAT. In this slightly cropped length, this evergreen coat can look very charming.

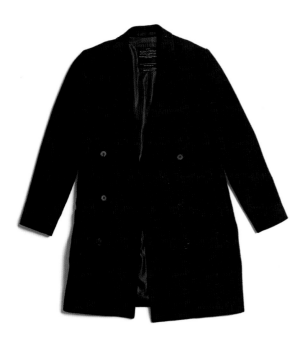

A CLASSIC BLACK MENSWEAR OVERCOAT. Whether single or double-breasted, this piece will elevate anything else you're wearing—yes, even your most beat-up jeans.

A CLASSIC CAMEL WOOL OVERCOAT. This shade looks superrich and particularly chic with just a white shirt and jeans (especially white jeans).

The Timeless Classic: A Peacoat

Even pieces like regulation navy peacoats, striped shirts, and simple white jeans can look unique if you accent them the right way. Everything Caroline is wearing is classic and will always be in style, but it also has a certain cool factor: the pants have a wide flare, and the jacket fits just right—it's not too boxy or shrunken. And with the bandana (one of the most classic pieces there is), the outfit comes together to create an easy, timeless, hip-girl look.

"My peacoat is the one I go for over and over. It makes everything look cool without being overly trendy. It never gets old."

—Caroline Forsling

The Kooky Classic: A Leopard-Print Coat

Leopard print, velvet, black sequins (gold and silver get too flashy), beads, pony hair, subtle ruffles, lace, faux-fur jackets, and paisley can all look classically chic and not dated as long as the cut and the pairing is right. Janis, who does "sexy classic" so well, throws this leopard-print coat over simple pencil skirts and trousers when she wants to stand out a bit.

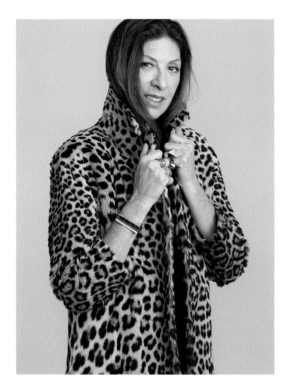

"It belonged to my mother, who gave it to me twenty years ago. It was a maxi coat that she cut short (too bad!). She stopped wearing it because people on the street always commented on it."

—Janis Savitt

The Euro-Chic Classic: The Trench Coat

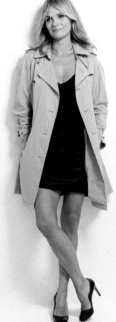

SEXY. Wearing a trench sexes up a simple slip dress with pumps, giving it a hint of sass without the tart factor. Keep it short like the dress—as Tina does here—for the cleanest silhouette.

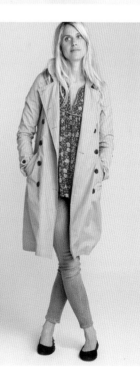

BOHO POLISHED. Throw a longer, men's-style trench over a full-on hippie look like Molly does. It keeps the trench from looking too serious and elevates the jeans.

ANATOMY OF

The Perfect Trench Coat

If you invest in a good trench coat, you can wear it forever. Burberry's is the prototype for what a classic piece should look like. If you're more into darker colors, try one in black. A trench coat makes anything you're wearing underneath it look that much more polished, and it's just really so versatile.

When shopping for a classic trench, you'll want to keep a few key points in mind.

PIPED SEAMS ON THE INSIDE are a refined detail.

A REMOVABLE LINING IS GREAT FOR COLDER WEATHER but not a requisite.

A SLIM SET-IN SLEEVE CREATES THE CHICEST ARM SILHOUETTE.

WRIST BELTS THAT MATCH THE MAIN ONE ARE KEY.

EPAULETS ARE A MUST-HAVE EMBELLISHMENT—even though they serve no modern purpose!

A FRONT "GUN" FLAP LOOKS COOL. (It was originally designed to keep rain from penetrating.)

DOUBLE-BREASTED IS THE MOST CLASSIC CUT. Although if you feel slimmer in a single-breasted style, go for it.

A BELT WITH A STITCHED LEATHER-COVERED BUCKLE IS A RICH-LOOKING DETAIL—a million times better than plastic or metal.

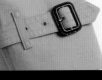

GOOD BUTTONS ARE VITAL. The most luxe option is imitation bone.

Make a Hippie Outfit Classically French

I love mixing boho and classic, like a flowy dress with a blazer, a drapey kimono (short or long) over a simple outfit, or a tough-looking leather jacket with floaty pants. It makes everything cooler and more relaxed. To wit: Molly always wears Indian tops with her jeans, which can be misconstrued as, well, too hippie-dippy. But she always adds the right accessories—classic, girlie, or preppy pieces like top-handled handbags or a sharp jacket—that take this look somewhere less crunchy. Slip on French-style ballet flats and the outfit goes from "Grateful Dead groupie" to "Left-Bank Parisian."

More Pieces That Add Polish

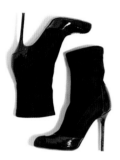

SHOES like high-heeled, sexy ankle boots (remember the skinny ankle silhouette!); ballet flats; sneakers (classic Converse or Adidas—no running or aerobics shoes); or lace-up men's oxfords.

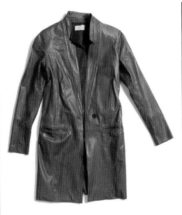

A TAILORED MEN'S-STYLE DUSTER-LENGTH LEATHER OR WOOL COAT that hits a few inches below the knee.

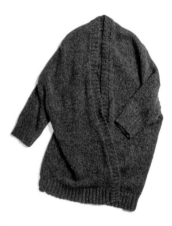

A COZY CASHMERE CARDIGAN. Adding something so luxe makes any boho piece seem tony.

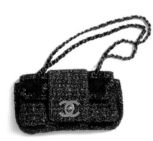

A DESIGNER BAG with rich details like subtle gold or silver hardware and chain straps. (Chanel, of course, but you can also fake it—so many less-expensive designers like Kate Spade and Rebecca Minkoff make similar good-looking ones that tell the same story.)

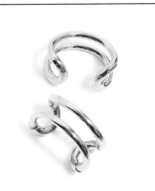

BOLD GOLD JEWELRY like a strong cuff or bangle (it doesn't have to be real!), big hoops, or a cigar-band ring can't be beat for elevating a look.

TIP: One classic piece is all you need to tone down the funk.

Getting the Most Out of Your Wardrobe

Use Bohemian Pieces to Cool Up the Classics

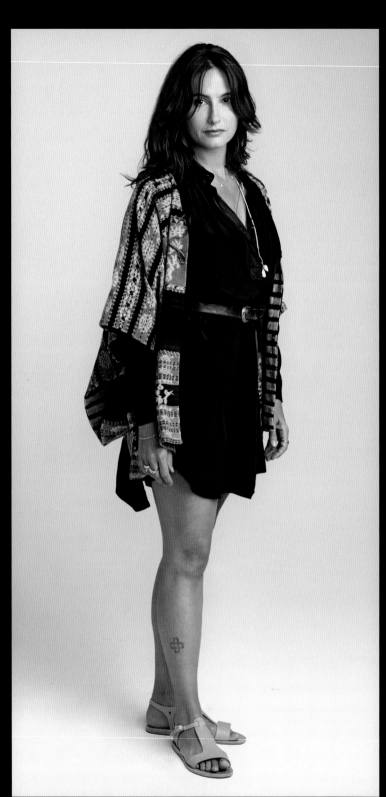

ARTSY. Scosha always adds at least one boho piece to her overall look. By layering a short vintage kimono over a simple shirtdress, she transforms it into something a bit more hippie-ish.

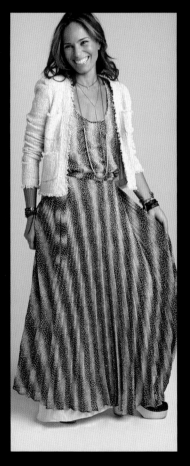

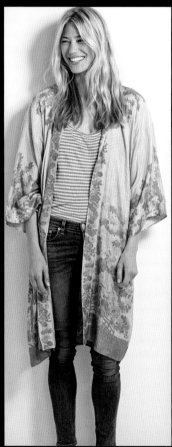

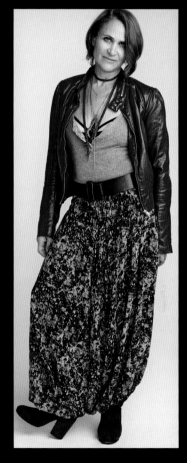

UPPER-CRUST. A classic bouclé jacket can read too "lady." But Kaela wears it over a long, flowy dress for a touch of boho.

ECLECTIC. Caroline turns an ordinary jeans-and-tee ensemble into a personal style manifesto. All she did was don a soft vintage kimono (with no rips or stains—always key) over a boyish striped tee and skinny jeans, which on their own are cute but tell a much plainer story.

EDGY. From the waist up, Susan is all casual in her tough leather-and-tee combo. Adding the somewhat wild flowing printed harem pants created a more boho vibe. I love that she anchored the whole thing with substantial urban booties.

Q&A with Anna Bakst, President of Michael Kors Accessories

Who are your style icons?

I think my environment is my biggest influence—seeing the inspiration boards for the season, what people are wearing in the office, and what's going on on the streets of New York (I live downtown).

What are the items in your closet that you've had the longest and will never throw out?

I am obsessed with jackets and jeans, and some novelty T-shirts bring back memories. I also keep my outerwear. I'm glad I've kept these items, as I still pull out some of my older jackets. The jeans don't fit the same way they did back then.

What is your favorite body part to emphasize?

My head/face. People can get a sense of who you are through your facial expressions and eyes.

What was your first fashion splurge and why?

Calvin Klein jeans. The Brooke Shields ad was the inspiration. That was a very big purchase. I grew up in Champaign, Illinois, and there wasn't much fashion going on there.

What are your favorite accessories?

My wedding band. I like it!

Any signature beauty or hair thing you do?

I get a keratin treatment every six months to reduce frizz; this way I can let my hair dry naturally and it keeps things very low maintenance. And yes, I do get my hair colored to cover the grays.

Do you only have expensive designer clothing or do you mix?

Mix! One of my favorite shirts is a denim shirt from Kmart—it's the best!

Do you have any fashion pet peeves?

I like things to last. I tend to wear what I like over and over again, so the quality needs to be there to some degree. I prefer jeans with little to no stretch—I have to work hard to find good jeans today as so many have a lot of it. APC pre-worn jeans are a good go-to with no stretch.

Name some fashion rules you live by.

Not sure about any rules—they may exist subconsciously. But here is what is consistent about me: If you love it, wear it! Don't worry about preserving it or the opposite, how many times people have seen you in it. Wear what you love! In the end it's you that comes through, not the clothes. And finally, a smile is the best accessory.

Name five things you think every woman should have in her closet.

Sexy black heels, a tuxedo jacket, relaxed jeans, a perfect white T-shirt, and a white dress shirt.

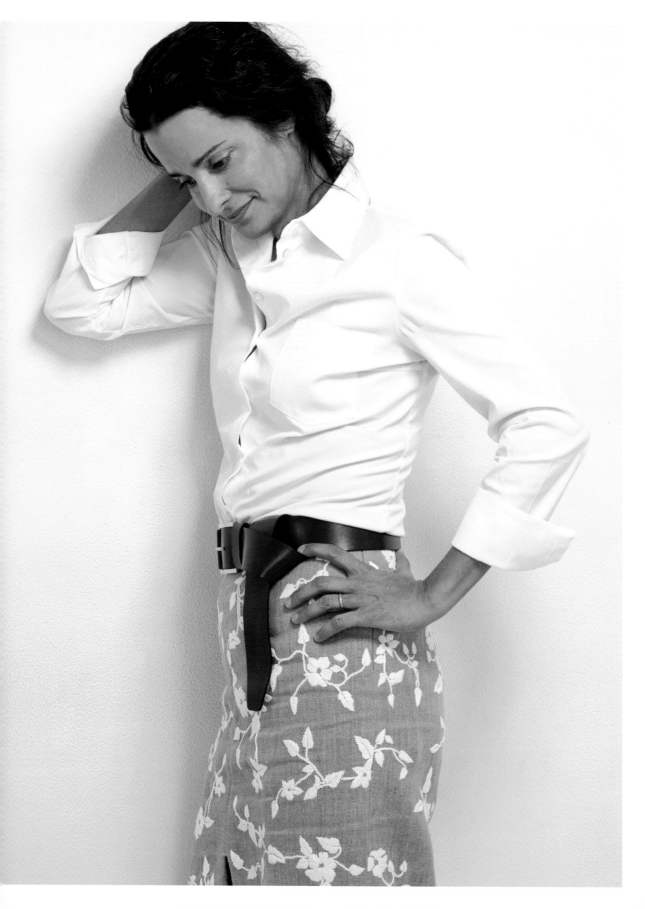

DRESSING IN BLACK AND WHITE ISN'T SO BLACK-AND-WHIT

These two colors (or noncolors) have long been synonymous with effortless urban chic, probably because they're hard to mess up. Black and white pieces are closet staples. They look good on almost everyone and are versatile enough for any situation. A good white button-down and pair of classic black trousers can be worn in so many ways.

The challenge is to mix and match these practical shades without looking like a cater waiter, a phenomenon I've encountered far too often. I'll teach you how to get the balance just right. And I promise that with a little guidance, you can wear these colors monochromatically—a shortcut to looking chic—without coming across as a member of a religious cult or a Bauhaus groupie. A great finishing touch in every case can be a dash of color; note that neutrals like gray and camel can have as big an impact as bold brights.

The Right Balance Is Critical

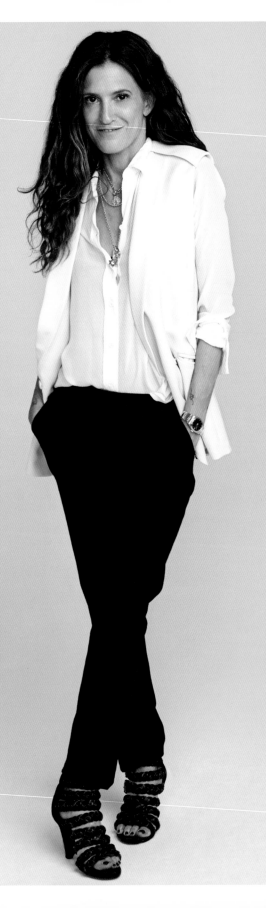

It's so easy to get this wrong and look more like a waitperson than a chic and sophisticated woman. The problem is usually not the pieces themselves but how they're assembled. Off the runway, even the coolest black trousers—a pair of Ann Demeulemeesters, say—worn with a black blazer and a white button-down can come across as more service uniform than high-style suit. The solution, thankfully, is simple.

When you're feeling too uniform-y, swap a plain white shirt for something with more presence. And if you're going for a tuxedo look, a classic pleated or ruffle-front shirt is great.

Another option: by keeping the tops all the same shade (like I do here), you get instant chic, not boring or institutional. The same works with a black top and jacket plus white or ecru pants—which I wear all year long. Style knows no season, after all.

I love a white blazer with a same-color T-shirt or blouse; choose black pants to ground the outfit.

ALL-WEATHER WHITES. Here's an unconventionally great example of how white pants work year-round: Susan pairs a chunky black turtleneck sweater with softer, billowy white pants and slim heels that balance the baggy silhouette. The result is a modern-day, downtown riff on Katharine Hepburn cool.

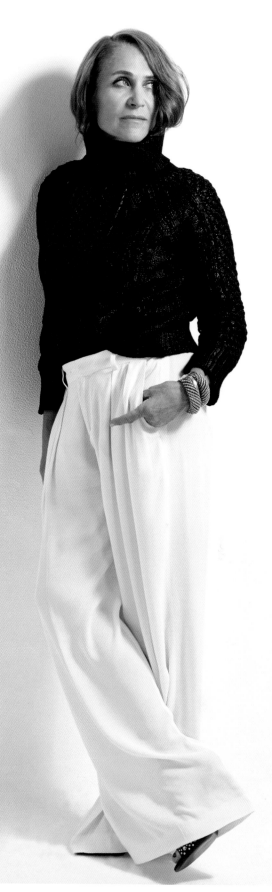

4 Ways to Pull Off Head-to-Toe Black

All-black can be read in so many ways: fancy or casual, feminine or tomboyish, artsy— or just plain cool.

I. **DRESSY.** Texture and shine give an all-black outfit the oomph it needs. A slinky Lurex top like April's, lamé, sequins, and black-on-black embroidery are all great choices. Mixing fabrics lends interest and dimension; even nubby wool can add texture and break up the monotony, thereby making everything look richer. Same goes for little extras like pleats and ruffles.

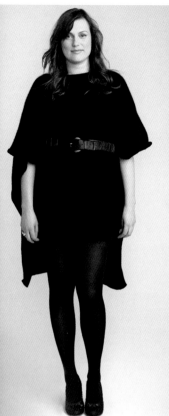

2. ARTSY. Leigh's vintage look is dramatic because of the shape of the cape dress: those batwing sleeves *make* the outfit. And she keeps everything—tights, belt, shoes—opaque black. Even the tailoring is perfect: the high neck balances the short length. High/low is always the way to go.

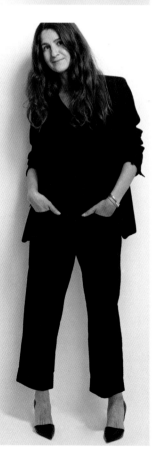

3. MINIMAL. Courtesy of its strong, edgy silhouette, Laura's slightly boxy black jumpsuit/jacket combo reads downtown chic. (Jumpsuits are always a little funky in and of themselves.) Laura opts for Birkenstocks when she's running around the set all day, but here, the pointy-toed pumps add a little urban-tough glamour.

4. FEMININE. Juxtaposing a flash of skin with ladylike accessories makes for a soft and pretty look. Lisa unbuttoned her amazing vintage dress low, belted it, rolled up the sleeves, and kept her legs bare. (Lacy or refined fishnet hosiery also would've worked.) With sexy ankle boots and a strand of pearls, she realized a flirty, somewhat sexy '70s feeling—making her dress look like classic YSL. And I love that her pearls are black, not white.

TIP: To keep your black pieces looking their darkest, wash them in cold water and don't toss them in the dryer. That said, if pieces *do* fade, don't ditch them: they can look super cool paired with darker blacks. I love a faded, almost-gray black tee with dark, dark black skinny jeans and boots.

Black Looks Great with Blue or Gray, and Even a Pop of Red

One of my all-time favorite combinations, both sophisticated and unexpected, is black with navy or a more nuanced and bohemian indigo. The shades are similar enough that they meld together instead of cutting you in half.

I also love mixing in neon brights and primary shades like acid yellow, cherry red, and electric blue.

Daryl goes for a pop of red with her cool, somewhat ironic fanny pack and fun biker jacket.

CONTEMPORARY TWIST. April's black-on-black jacket/top combo sets off her light-gray trousers, giving them an edgy presence (unlike a navy or gray blazer would) and creating a mismatched suit that feels less cookie-cutter than the norm. Pants with an extra-large silhouette look even more modern.

TIP: If you're not comfortable going this slouchy, try a more moderate menswear-style pant that sits right at the hip.

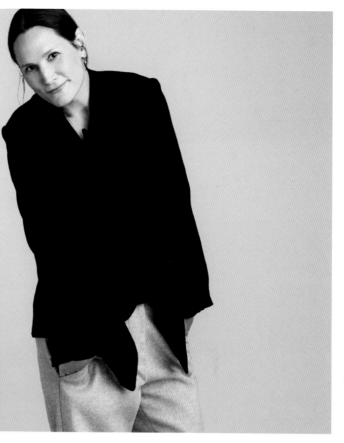

THE ANTI-UNIFORM. Here, Leigh mixes moods. Her otherwise sporty navy tee makes the serious black pencil skirt look laid-back, whereas all black would veer toward workplace-serious or channel a cocktail waitress. The navy pumps elevate the outfit, making it more interesting than obvious black would.

TIP: You'll never be able to match blacks exactly unless you buy a black suit, but that's OK: layering in texture and a nice dark heather gray or rich brown will pull them together.

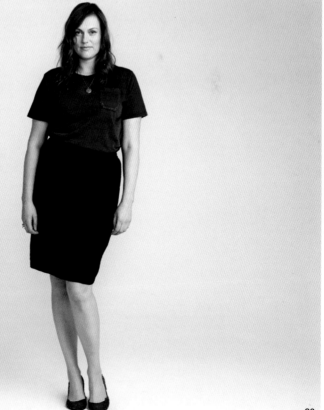

How to Pull Off Head-to-Toe White

An all-white outfit is so elemental and clean, especially in the heat of the summer. Not to mention, it's one of the easiest ways to get dressed. One of my favorite classic looks is white jeans and a white tee with sand-colored Arizona Birkenstocks—a bit boho but still sharp. But all-white can also be super feminine, or even a little rock 'n' roll.

And I know it sounds funny, but just remember to carry Shout Wipes in your bag. Nothing works better on spills. (That Tide pen doesn't come close!)

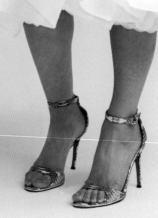

FEMININE. Anamaria layers the same stark-white shade to create a skirt suit that looks like a crisp and girlie 1940s summer dress.

ROCK 'N' ROLL. Daryl's all-white look is more punky. The silk blouse, leather skirt, and platform Birkenstocks get a dose of bad-boy chic thanks to her signature black-leather biker hat.

Not Quite All-White, but Still the Same Effect

You don't need to wear full-on super-optical white to achieve this clean, monochromatic look. Another option is to mix white with shades that are close approximates: a tinge of a pastel color (like pink or the palest yellow) or an off-white like cream, wheat, or ecru. Here's how to look fresh without wearing top-to-bottom white.

A MATCHUP OF CREAM AND WHITE.
Creating a mismatched suit with different milky tones works when you keep the top lighter than the bottom, or vice versa.

How to Turn Summer Whites into Cool Bohemian Looks

Whites can feel earthy when you add the right warm accessories, like sandals, wrist cuffs, and a satchel in natural, olive, or dark-brown leather or suede.

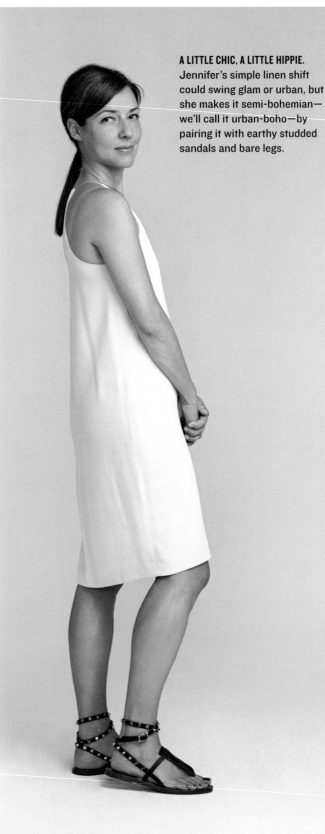

A LITTLE CHIC, A LITTLE HIPPIE. Jennifer's simple linen shift could swing glam or urban, but she makes it semi-bohemian— we'll call it urban-boho—by pairing it with earthy studded sandals and bare legs.

RELAXED ELEGANCE. Gayle's cool dress is actually a vintage nightshirt, which she collects. (Search for Edwardian and Victorian cotton ones on eBay or Etsy and at flea markets.) Her slightly patinated vintage hunting saddle bag and natural leather high-heeled A Détacher sandals make her look Euro, like she's running around Barcelona in July.

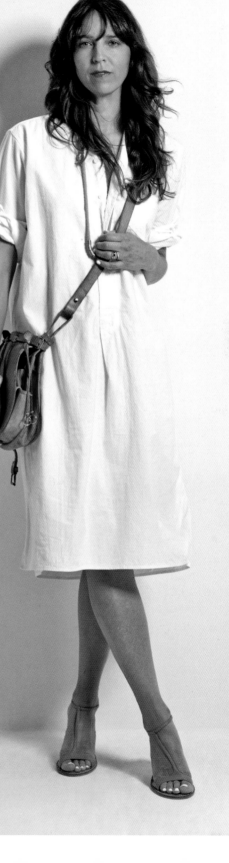

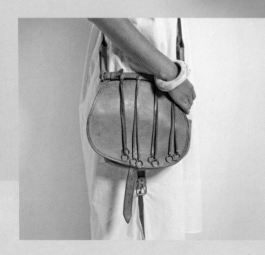

ANATOMY OF
The Perfect Tee

The right T-shirt can be worn so many ways: with pencil skirts and heels, menswear trousers, and—of course—jeans. A good fabric and cut will take you anywhere. When you find the perfect version, buy a few backups so you can keep them in maximum rotation. Here are the features to look for.

NECK. The crew neck should be a tiny bit loose, hitting at or slightly below the clavicle. If it isn't, just stretch it out by hand. If it's a V-neck, make sure the point of the V doesn't stop too high or too low: four inches from the start of your clavicle is good (the perfect length for showing off necklaces on skin).

FIT. A tee should fit you the way it fits a guy: not too loose, not skintight—especially around the torso and chest.

A GOOD-WEIGHT FABRIC. It shouldn't be too thick (like a Beefy-T) or thin (steer clear of sheer). Look for Japanese cotton, which hangs classically—like a really worn-in man's undershirt. When in doubt, try J. Crew.

CLASSIC COLORS OTHER THAN WHITE. Tees in black, navy, and heather gray are all great. (Just make sure to get the right heather gray: too light looks cheap. Look for a mix of poly to channel that good gray from old gym tees and sweats.)

SLEEVES. They should extend three or four inches from the shoulder and be snug enough so as to not bag too wide around the arm. Rolling them up is another option. I also love a narrow sleeve that hits just above the elbow—very Jane Birkin. And if you hate showing your arms altogether, consider a slouchy long-sleeved tee with slightly loose arms. Then roll them up to just under the elbow.

LENGTH. A tee should hit about two inches below your hipbone—just long enough to half tuck it in the front.

Getting the Most Out of Your Wardrobe

An Ode to the Jumpsuit

This one-piece wonder has gone in and out of fashion for years, but I believe it's finally here to stay. It's a great dress alternative (especially for those of us who don't love our legs). Insta-style! And lest you think there's only one look you can achieve, check out all of these. The game changers here are shoes and belts. Think outside the box to make this piece yours.

"The jumpsuit is one piece: done! For me, it's also a no-fail. You can wear jumpsuits casually with sneakers or cuffed with your highest heels. They're sexy without clinging to the body. For that same reason, you can fit great lingerie underneath; I take every opportunity to wear my favorite vintage bodysuits: a peek of some beautiful lace in the neckline or through the button placket never ruined anyone's day."

Christina Kornilakis

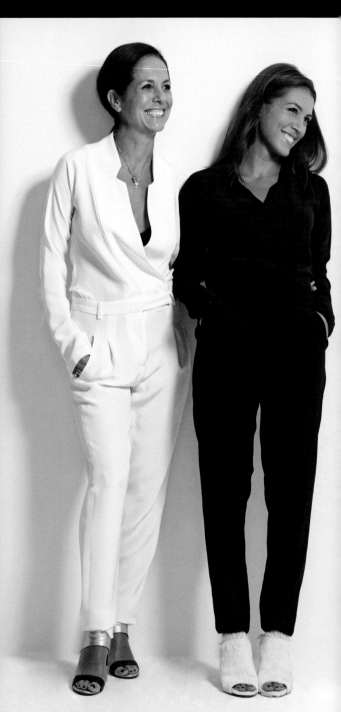

Jumpsuits can be super sleek, as in the case of Maria and her daughter, Bibi. Maria's is almost like a suit, kept minimal with an interesting bare shoe, while Bibi (in black) shocks the eye with white pony slides.

Susan loves jumpsuits for her everyday work uniform: they're easy and effortless, with maximum comfort when you're on your feet all day. She rolls up the sleeves, unbuttons it low to reveal all of her necklaces, and tucks the hems into cool bohemian boots.

Christina makes a plain white mechanic's jumpsuit chic by unbuttoning the front down to the waist and revealing a pretty teddy underneath. High-heeled wedge Mary Janes sweeten the look.

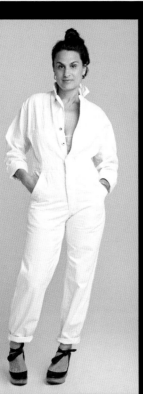

Gayle goes for a super-baggy military flight suit, which she scored at a flea market. She cinches the waist and adds strappy heels for a way-sexy look. Note: it's hard to find a vintage jumpsuit that fits perfectly; have a tailor take the legs in and raise the crotch if needed.

Q&A with Kim Gordon, Rock Star, Artist, and Writer

What was your first fashion splurge and why?

A pair of red corduroy hip-hugger bell-bottoms that I bought in Hong Kong when I was twelve. It was an English colony then and this one store carried mod clothes.

Who are your style icons?

Anita Pallenberg, Françoise Hardy.

Describe your beauty routine, including products used.

Rodin face oil, Kiehl's coconut shampoo, Chanel light foundation, Oribe hair spray.

How would you describe your style? How has it evolved over the years?

Tomboy lite. I used to wear a lot of band T-shirts.

What are the items in your closet that you've had the longest and will never throw out?

Pink sequined Miu Miu shoes.

Who are your favorite designers?

Acne jeans and boots are great. Dresses are easy— Saint Laurent for classics, Rodarte for pure beauty, Marc Jacobs for wild imagination mixed with femininity.

Foolproof work outfit?

Silver glitter shoes I did with Surface to Air, sequined Phillip Lim shorts, and a T-shirt.

Is there anything you wear every single day?

Gold safety-pin earrings.

Is there anything you do that breaks conventional fashion rules?

I probably shouldn't be wearing shorts onstage.

What is your definition of cool style?

Not cheesy, or cutesy, or trying too hard.

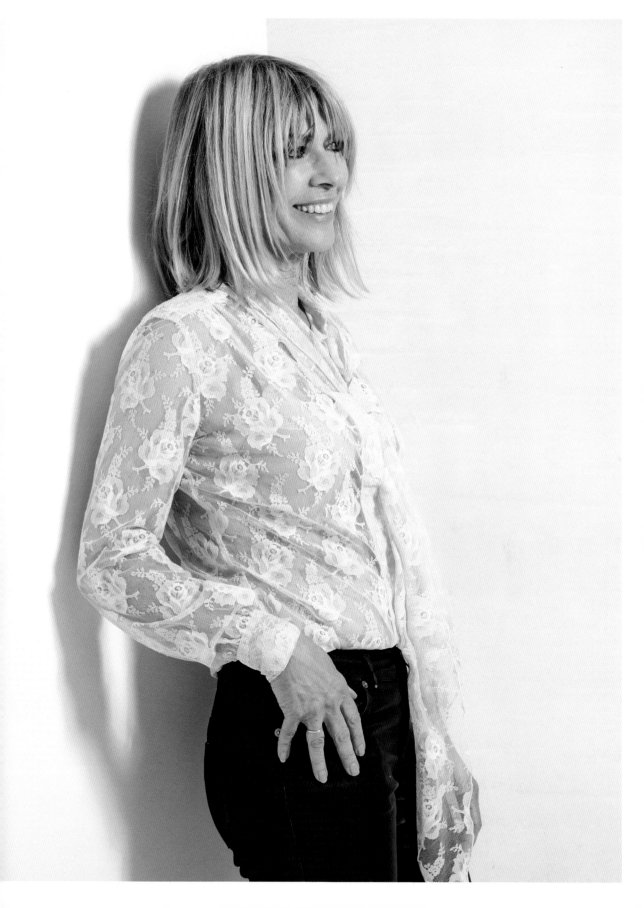

PSSST!
LAYERING IS THE SECRET TO PERSONA STYLE

How many times have you seen a woman with great style pull off a miraculous layering trick—that uncanny ability of knowing what looks good over and under everything? Sure, we all know to wear a tank top under a sheer blouse to combat the see-through effect, or to throw a sweater over a long-sleeved T-shirt to stay warm. But imaginative, strategic layering is what makes all the difference when it comes to cool.

Luckily, you probably already have everything you need to become a master layerer hanging in your closet and tucked into your drawers. Thin long-sleeved tees, snug and oversize jackets, thin turtlenecks, and even full-length slips are all ripe for throwing on top of one another. The secret is knowing what works together.

Surprise, Surprise! You Can Even Layer Jackets

I've always layered jackets as a means to feel and look chicer (and because I tend to run cold). For this to work, the one underneath has to be cut a bit trimmer and made from a fabric thin enough so that it slips cleanly under the one on top and doesn't bunch up in the armpits. I love wearing denim jackets under blazers to create a casual effect (that's also warm). The skinny belt adds interest and creates a nice waistline, so the layered jackets don't look too bulky.

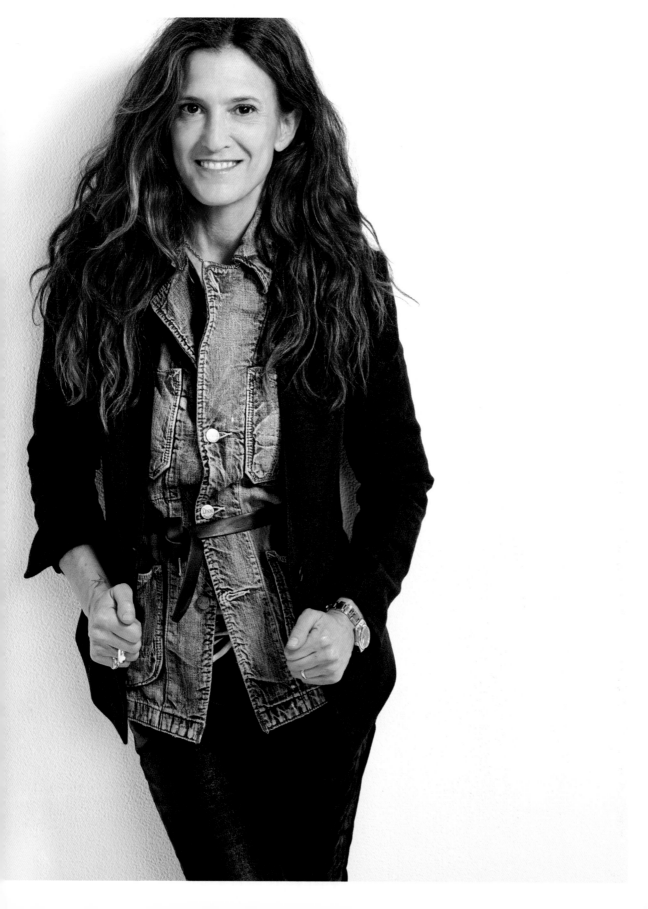

These are some easy, at-hand pieces that layer like a charm.

A-List Layering Pieces

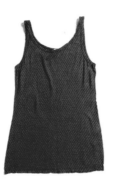

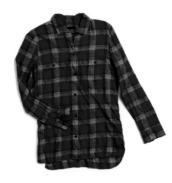

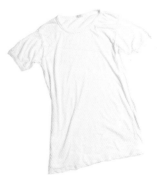

TANK TOP. Wear one under pretty much anything—for warmth, of course, but also to lend interest. Let the straps peek out of a wider neckline or the hem out of the bottom of a shirt or sweater. Use tanks to add a pop of color or contrast underneath a sheer top. Layering two tank tops looks even more interesting; the one underneath should ideally be longer so it hangs out a little, and so the fabrics lie better.

MENSWEAR BUTTON-DOWN SHIRT. Great worn over a thin turtleneck with the sleeves rolled up and a few buttons undone à la the final scene in Annie Hall. Toss an outsize cardigan or blazer on top for extra coziness.

T-SHIRT. Wear a short-sleeved tee over a more formfitting long-sleeved one to achieve a cool tomboy spirit that will also keep you much warmer during wintertime.

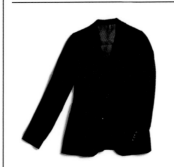

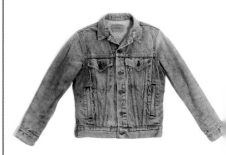

BLAZER. Be creative and use this buttoned-up workplace staple in a casual or festive manner—over a sequined cardigan that's layered atop a silk shell, for instance.

DENIM JACKET. This versatile piece will undercut the stuffiness of whatever it's paired with, even a structured jacket or coat.

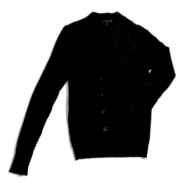

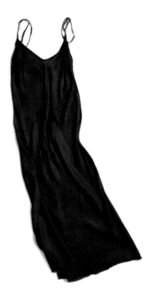

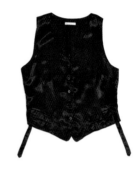

THIN OR CHUNKY V-NECK CARDIGAN. You can layer these over almost any top—and under any jacket. Cinch with a skinny belt and you'll be the chicest woman in the room. Go for a fitted cardie or a thicker baggy version over another piece.

SLIP DRESSES AND CAMISOLES. A slip dress layered over a T-shirt equals a casual daytime look; pair the outfit with sneakers, ankle boots, or sandals. Wearing a short slip over a longer one creates a nice tiered effect. You can also opt for a long camisole, even one with a lace hem that peeks out. (I'm a sucker for pretty things intentionally dangling.)

MEN'S-STYLE VEST. I love to slip one of these under a blazer paired with jeans, elevating the outfit to a dandyish level. Vests also layer perfectly over slip dresses, imparting an unexpectedly masculine vibe. Try both a fitted and a roomier version.

TIP: Whether the vest is loose or snug, its armholes shouldn't ever gape out at the sides (an easy fix at the tailor, where he can nip the sides in).

5 Steps to Chic and Warm

There's a stylish way to layer for warmth without creating unflattering bulk or feeling like a sausage. Lisa demonstrates a perfectly put-together outfit.

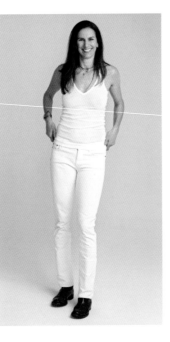

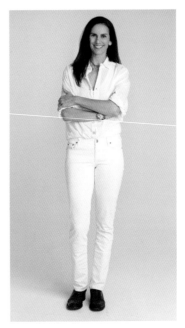

I. BASE LAYER. Lisa went for white jeans and a simple white cotton tank. Blue jeans and a black tank—or trousers and a silk camisole—are nice alternatives.

2. A THIN LAYER FOR WARMTH. Here, she chose a classic menswear white button-down. Let the first layer peek through: yes, it's functional, but it's also part of the outfit, so exploit the opportunity.

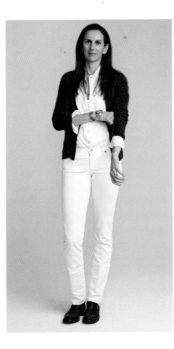

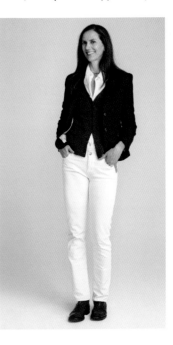

3. A LIGHTWEIGHT, FITTED V-NECK CARDIGAN. Fasten a few buttons only.

4. A LITTLE BLAZER. You can remove it (or the cardigan) if needed. A blazer nonchalantly perched on the shoulders always looks cool, too.

5. COAT AND HAT. Toss on your outerwear, and voilà: überfunctional yet totally chic.

4 Steps to a More Interesting Outfit

A jumpsuit isn't the most obvious or seemingly practical choice for a base layer. Even on its own, it's a tricky piece to wiggle in and out of (especially in the loo). But it works wonderfully as a layering element. Choose one that slides off the shoulders so it's easier to slip off; if you pick one that opens in the front, you can shrug off all the layers in a single gesture. Take cues from how Caroline does it.

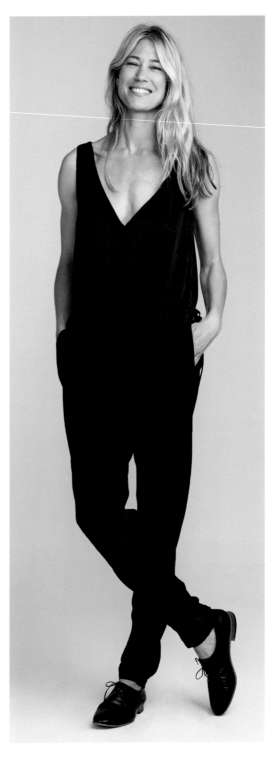

I. SILK JUMPSUIT. Caroline's base is an easy-yet-polished piece of her own design that she conceived to be worn myriad ways: alone in summer, layered for fall.

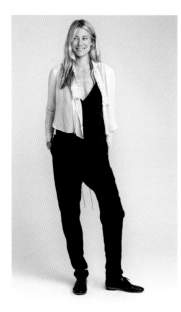

2. VICTORIAN BLOUSE. Next, she adds an antique cotton-and-lace top. Pieces like this, with beautiful handmade lace or crocheted trim, are easily found in flea markets and on eBay and Etsy. (Search "Victorian" or "Edwardian" and make sure the item is pristine, without holes or stains.)

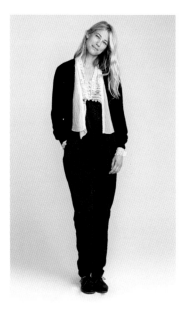

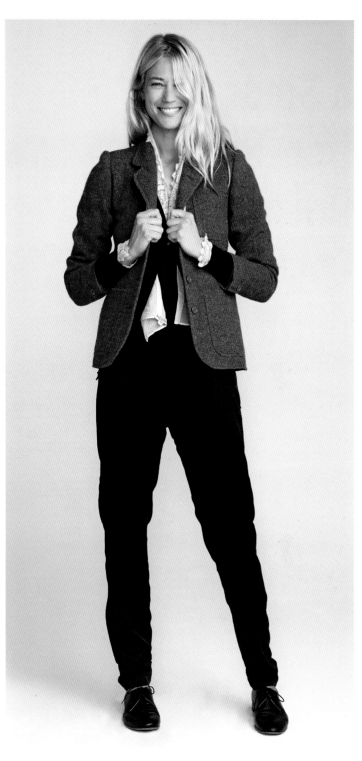

3. MIDWEIGHT CARDIGAN. A simple merino wool or cashmere sweater comes next. In this case, a V-neck was essential to showcase the blouse's lace collar.

4. SHRUNKEN TWEED BLAZER. Caroline's is a vintage YSL, but so many labels—from Theory to Mango—make good ones, season after season.

5 Steps from Slip Dress to Complete Outfit

A slip dress is like a blank canvas for your creativity. Layer pieces under or over it—or both. It's such a simple and versatile garment, and so chameleon-like: it can read as a skirt when you cover up the top or as a work-appropriate dress when worn with a jacket or a streamlined sweater. Turn a simple silk-charmeuse version (long or knee-length) into a full-on cool outfit by adding these pieces.

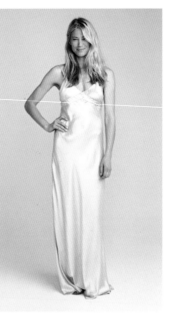

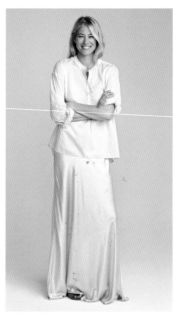

I. A SIMPLE SLIP. Super versatile and a great layering base, slips can be found in lingerie shops. Choose a good style for your body type; avoid a bias cut if you're worried about saddlebags.

2. A SOFT WHITE BLOUSE. Loose and poetic, this imparts a romantic feel. Choosing the same color as the slip keeps the effect long and lean.

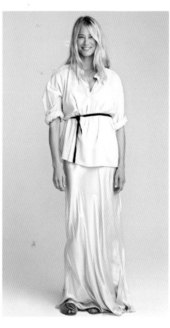

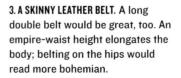

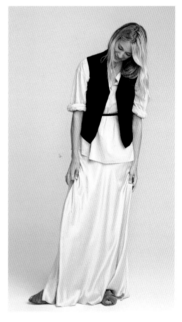

3. A SKINNY LEATHER BELT. A long double belt would be great, too. An empire-waist height elongates the body; belting on the hips would read more bohemian.

4. A FITTED MENSWEAR VEST. It adds an element of quirky masculinity.

5. AN OVERSIZE DUSTER. A tailored menswear coat would work, too— really, anything short of a down parka or a rain slicker.

Layer Your Way to Individuality

Christene always dresses to the beat of her own drum, and her fun layering combinations are an integral facet of her look. She piles them on not for warmth so much as to have fun with patterns and textures—and to showcase her signature eclectic style. And yes, there's a method to her madness.

- **CHOOSE WIDE-LEG PANTS.** A long slip under a shorter dress is the failsafe choice. But Christene thinks outside the box with a flowy pair of gauchos—pants with a skirtlike quality. The combination not only looks fresh, it's also practical, rendering dress-wearing more comfy.

- **MIX MOTIFS FEARLESSLY.** Even stripes, plaids, and florals can live harmoniously with a little trial and error. Here, Christene pairs a classic menswear plaid with two types of stripes: a skinny vertical one and a wide sailor stripe.

- **FIND A CONSTANT.** Christene's bronze metallic shoes tie into the subtle stripe in her dress.

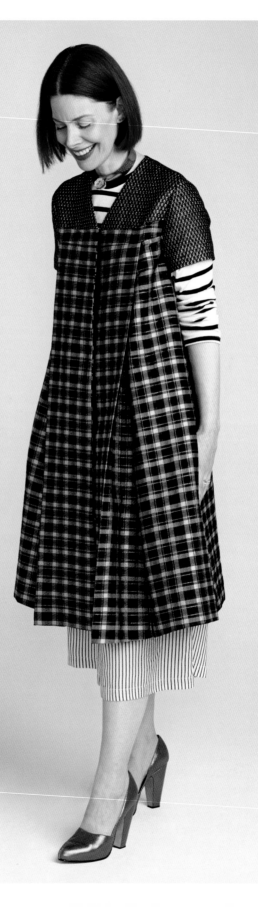

Layering Patterns That Seem to Clash but Actually Work Well Together

- Larger plaids like black watch or classic tartan and smaller checks

- Checks and polka dots

- Polka dots and stripes

- Stripes and florals

- Florals and plaids, polka dots, or checks

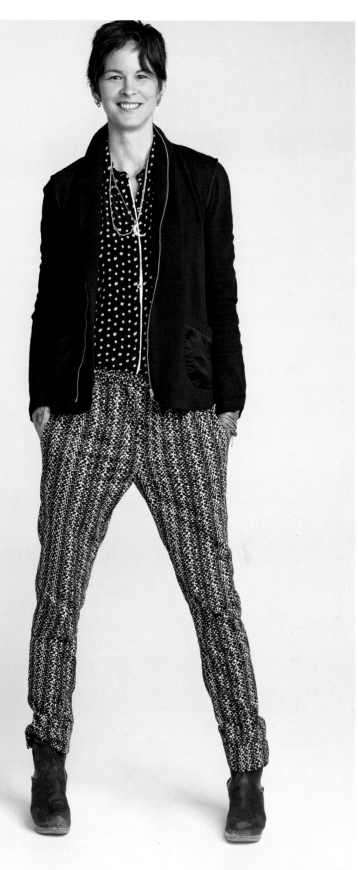

Michele's pattern mixing works without looking like she's trying too hard. Why? The polka-dot top and slightly ethnic pants are both in complementary blues and whites, which makes the patterns blend seamlessly. Finally, the solid jacket in a similar shade ties it all together.

Layering Math: Season by Season

Simple everyday pieces add up to so much more when they're mixed to produce unexpected combinations.

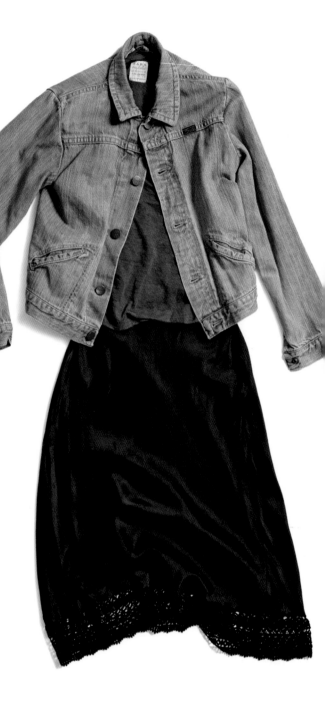

SPRING: Slip with long-sleeved tee and shrunken denim jacket

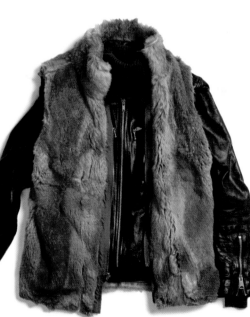

FALL: Striped long-sleeved tee with a denim shirt and a sleeveless blazer

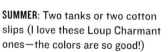

SUMMER: Two tanks or two cotton slips (I love these Loup Charmant ones—the colors are so good!)

WINTER: Leather jacket over a warm turtleneck with a furry vest over everything

ANATOMY OF

The Perfect Button-Down

A good men's-style shirt can be layered in so many ways. Consider these attributes when shopping for the right one—the subtleties will make a difference between a good-enough shirt and a great one that you'll use in a variety of combos. It may seem laborious, but you'll thank me later.

A NON-BUTTON-DOWN COLLAR, which can feel too specifically preppy.

NO STAYS in the collar—although a tailor can always remove them if you find a good vintage one that has them.

NO DARTS. They scream "lady," and not in a good way.

PEARL BUTTONS in the same color as the shirt. If you find a black button-down that you love but the buttons don't match, have a tailor change them. There's nothing worse than a cheap-looking white plastic button on a dark shirt.

NO CONCEALED PLACKET. It's much more classic to flaunt your buttons!

AT LEAST TWO BUTTONS ON THE CUFF (and an extra one sewn on the inside in case you lose one).

A LONG TAIL rather than one that's cut straight across. It just looks more "borrowed from the boys."

A COLLAR THAT'S NEITHER TOO LONG AND POINTY NOR TOO ROUND. A tailor can help neutralize an exaggerated one.

A BREAST POCKET. It's more casual than no pocket (and it's not a bad idea to own both versions).

FABRIC THAT'S THIN ENOUGH to hang well but not at all sheer.

Former No-No's Become Yes-Yesses

Weird Matchups

So many style books preach crazy rules about what is and is not acceptable. But women with personal style make up their own rules because they truly know what works for them.

FUNNY TEES WITH SERIOUS SKIRTS. From the "things that aren't supposed to go together" files: Janis, who has a great sense of humor, loves her funny "I'm Very Very Happy" Moschino tee. Worn with a polished pencil skirt and heels, it's a cheeky statement for less-serious days or for weekends.

STRIPES AND STRIPES. I'm crazy about mixing things that you're not supposed to put together, like clashing colors (pink and red, anyone?) or different stripes, like Karen does here. This works because the stripes are the same weight and color but go two different ways: horizontal on top, vertical on the bottom. And she's also mixing the moods of the two pieces: a slightly classic sailor tee with the mildly punk-rock vibe of the pants.

Former No-No's Become Yes-Yesses

Night for Day

We all have pieces in our closet that we rarely wear because we've deemed them "fancy" and are saving them for a special occasion. It's time to dust these off and give them daytime play. Pair them with your favorite jeans, simple work trousers, and everyday leather boots.

Just look at Pascale in her cool silver-sequined top—perfectly appropriate for the office. These are such easy looks, and yet they convey that she really knows what she's doing.

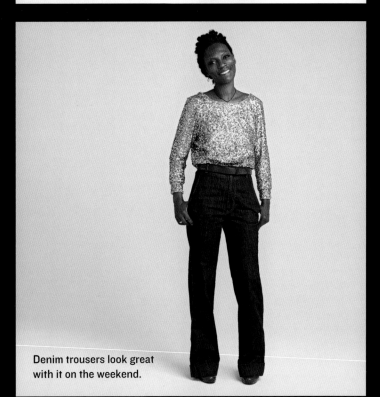

Add an A-line skirt and high-heeled Mary Janes for a work-to-party look.

Denim trousers look great with it on the weekend.

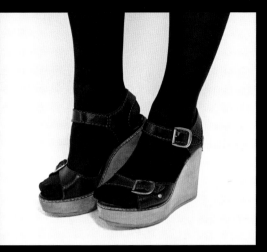

Socks with Sandals (or Fancy Shoes)

Sure, these shoes are great on their own with bare skin, but wearing them with simple kneesocks or polka-dot anklets can add instant fun. If you don't feel daring enough for the funkiness of a patterned sock, stick with a classic: midweight cashmere in a rich neutral like camel, gray, black, or navy is best and makes evening shoes look cool. Pick a color that matches the shoe to create the illusion of a formfitting ankle bootie (like Pascale does, bottom).

And it might sound obvious, but make sure your socks are in great shape (no holes or pilling) and that they don't get thinner and more sheer at the toe and heel—which sometimes happens when older socks stretch out. Consider buying a few pairs reserved just for the purpose of wearing with strappy and open-toed shoes.

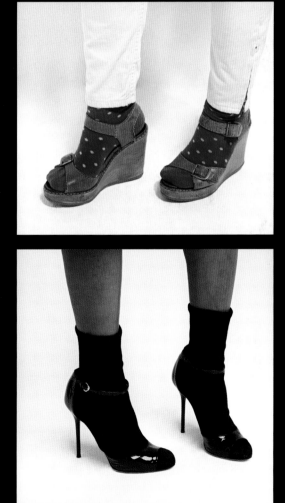

Q&A with Christene Barberich, Editor in Chief of Refinery29

What was your first fashion splurge and why?

A pair of black Gucci loafers that I bought at the flagship boutique on Madison Avenue in the mid '90s. I promised myself that when I finally became a published writer, I would go and buy myself a pair of Gucci loafers in the boutique. I was so young, so it cracks me up that *that* was the thing I wanted more than anything . . . really, a pair of loafers?

What are your go-to jeans? How do you usually style them?

Vintage high-waisted jeans, usually from the '70s—Wrangler tends to be my go-to brand on eBay. For contemporary jeans, it's Karen Walker and Rachel Comey.

Name some fashion rules you live by.

The only rule I believe in is being kind to others, as well as to yourself. Fashion is the antithesis of rules—everyone should be free to experience it and express themselves however they want to.

Go-to weekend outfit?

Workout clothes all day right into a crazy dress or trousers and a T-shirt with platforms and a long coat for dinner.

What did you used to wear all the time that you wouldn't dream of wearing now?

Flip-flops. I have a hard time even saying the word now.

What is your favorite body part to emphasize?

My neck. Ever since I read Nora Ephron's book *I Feel Bad About My Neck*, I moisturize my own like crazy.

What are your favorite accessories?

Heirloom jewelry and long gold pendants with a story behind them. I like jewelry with purpose and sentiment.

Do you have any fashion pet peeves?

It just makes me sad when I see people looking very obviously uncomfortable in their outfits, their shoes, their own skin. When you're comfortable, you just carry yourself more powerfully . . . and that's a wonderful, wonderful feeling.

Is there anything you've owned and worn for more than fifteen years?

A black cashmere Jil Sander cardigan. Every year I have these tiny holes repaired and keep on wearing it. It's beyond special.

Name five things you think every woman should have in her closet.

Again, it's different for every woman, but for me it would be white sneakers; pleated cropped black trousers; a long, dramatic printed coat; a great silky white shirt; and a bold piece of gold jewelry that makes me feel protected. I might even be wearing this very outfit today . . . wouldn't be the first time!

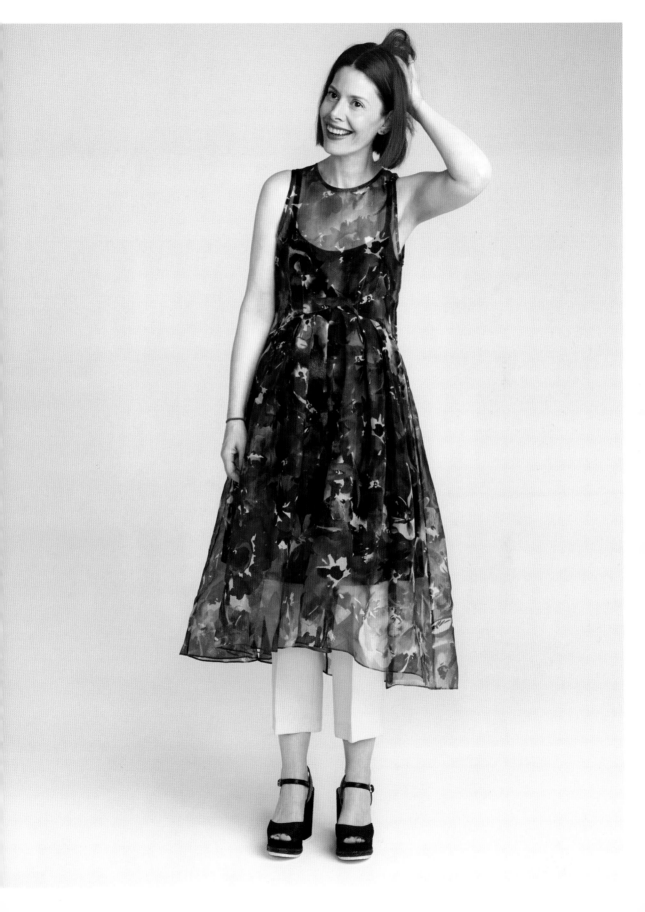

EVERYONE NEEDS A GOOD SUIT

No matter your personal style, nothing elevates your look like a suit. Trust me. Even when worn with Converse Chuck Taylors or a pair of combat boots, a suit conveys instant authority and polish. It is also a godsend in the morning: consider it a pre-matched outfit that offers no-brainer dressing with a built-in chic factor.

If the thought of a suit makes you break out in an anxious sweat, conjuring visions of corporate board meetings and stuffy offices, consider its many guises: there are feminine skirt suits, fierce skinny menswear ones, and even edgy velvet rock-star versions. Who can deny the sex appeal of Saint Laurent's Le Smoking from the 1970s, or Bianca Jagger's awesome wide-leg white wedding suit, topped with a groovy floppy hat? *Everyone*—even women who live in jeans—needs a suit. But, as with everything else, to look effortlessly cool, you need to wear the right one, the right way.

Suits Don't Have to Be Staid

While the mere idea of a suit can seem too serious, it can look totally cool if you put it together right, with all the fun extras that give it personality. A work suit can be just as sexy, exciting, and empowering as a fun evening one—if it's styled properly. Take a look at how these three women defy the corporate cliché.

The Look: Soft and Feminine

Although Anamaria works in fashion and can get away with wearing pretty much whatever she wants (lucky!), there are days when she needs to look that much more professional. In these situations, she opts for a cool, feminine suit with a shot of old-school glamour.

WHY IT WORKS: Because simple is usually better. A mid-calf-length skirt is superchic and—in the right cut—reads more high-fashion than a knee-length version would. Plus, the strappy heels (no sensible pumps here!) keep dowdiness in check. Here, she loses the jacket and throws on a trench.

"I'm partial to suits because of the instant put-togetherness they offer."
—Anamaria Wilson

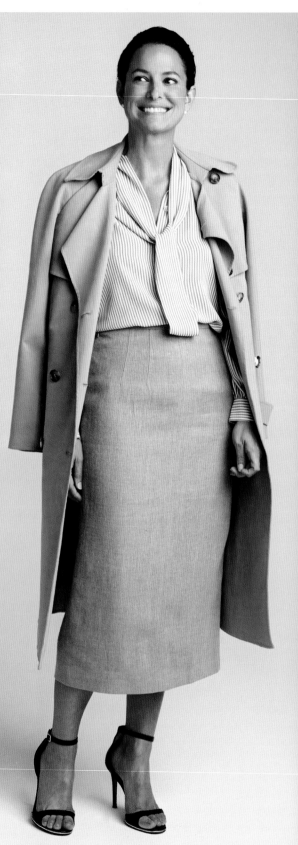

The Look:
Vintage Polish

Brooke rarely dresses conventionally and is adept at both mixing patterns and scoring mint-condition vintage finds. Her idea of a great suit is one that's modern but slightly retro.

WHY IT WORKS: The suit is vintage-y but not dated. A pop of color enlivens the otherwise monochromatic ensemble. Brooke anchors the pairing with a funky, modern-shaped shoe and sculptural Jill Platner jewelry—much savvier than the expected grandma-y pearls or cameo.

"Suits are a lazy girl's best friend. You look pulled together the moment you slip one on. Suits command respect and make people think you know exactly what you're doing. On those days when you feel like you're swimming in the dark, put on a suit and the lights will automatically turn on."

—Brooke Williams

The Look: Casual Cool

Though as a ceramicist she spends most of her days sporting clay-splattered jeans and clog boots, Michele still appreciates the sleekness and ease of a suit now and then. Her choice is a slightly slouchy menswear style.

WHY IT WORKS: With a T-shirt and sneakers, this suit is almost as relaxed as a pair of jeans—and certainly the opposite of stuffy. Michele is tall and lean enough to pull off a boxy man's suit; most women aspiring to a menswear look should head to the men's or boy's department and then get the suit tailored to be a bit more figure flattering. But you don't have to be so literal since there are also many designers (Ralph Lauren, Ann Demeulemeester, Dries van Noten, and Martin Margiela, as well as the fast fashion brands) who "borrow from the boys" and cut menswear suiting for women's bodies.

"This is my version of a black-tie dress. I love this suit because despite the super-classic color and cut, there's a lot of ease and comfort in the drape and the way the sleeves open up. It's not stiff or boxy like some men's suits; indeed, it's somehow a bit feminine—but not in a girlie way. The sneakers up the comfort level."

—Michele Quan

CHEAT SHEET

Suit-Shopping

In addition to giving you confidence, a well-chosen suit makes a versatile wardrobe staple: you can wear it for a serious meeting, dress it down with a T-shirt and flip-flops, or dress it up to the nines. Just keep the following guidelines in mind.

MAKE SURE THE JACKET FITS WELL IN THE SHOULDERS. The seam shouldn't stray too far away from the outside edge of your shoulder. Also, avoid shoulder pads that create an exaggerated silhouette in favor of those that follow the natural shape of your body. In addition, your upper arm shouldn't bulge out farther than the pad; if it does, you need a bigger size. (Or a great tailor to let out the shoulder a tad, but that's one of the toughest alterations to get right.) If the shoulders are way too big or small, skip it.

LOOK FOR POCKETS AND SLEEVE BUTTONS THAT ACTUALLY OPEN. A suit jacket is always more covetable when it has pockets you can put your hands into and cuffs that unbutton, something I learned from classic Savile Row menswear—the gold standard of tailoring. Admittedly, the sleeve detail is primarily symbolic, a subtle sign of money well spent. But operable buttons are also necessary when you want to push up the sleeves or let a shirt cuff hang out. On a good jacket, the pockets will be stitched down so the buyer is first to use them—and hence won't have lost their shape from too many try-ons.

VERSATILE, SEASONLESS FABRICS ARE YOUR BEST BET. Look for things like tropical wool, which can be worn most of the year, and crepe gabardine and matte cotton velvet in neutral shades, which will take you from fall to spring and can be dressed up or down. Anything heavy will undoubtedly be too bulky or hot for everyday use. In the summer, I love seersucker and crisp white cotton.

STICK WITH A CLASSIC SHAPE. To get the most wear out of a suit, invest in flattering shapes that will stand the test of time: a slight boot-cut or straight-leg pant, a pencil or A-line skirt. The most timeless jacket is a menswear cut. Avoid exaggerated proportions. A shrunken jacket and superwide pants might look cute in the moment, but they'll soon seem passé. (Save the trends for bargain-store finds at Topshop, Zara, Mango, and Asos.)

BUY SEPARATES. A well-cut blazer and pants (or skirt) in complementary shades can make up a chic mismatched suit. The pairing should look deliberate: close enough in value, but not so close that all you notice is the color differential. A cream jacket with a wheat-colored pant, light gray with dark gray, and navy with black are examples of good matchups. Make sure the fabric types work together in terms of both overall feeling and weight—don't pair wool with linen, for instance. But at the same time, don't try to match the fabrics exactly, because it will be impossible.

TIP: Don't split up a suit too often. It's fine once in a while, but wearing the blazer or pants solo will wear out the fabric unevenly, ultimately rendering the pieces two different shades.

The Rule Breakers

"Suit dressing" can be translated in so many ways, from classic to edgy, each with its own set of rules. Time to write a few rules of your own—after all, that's what personal style is all about.

Case No. 1: Classic

Take a cue from Anna, who layers a lightweight coat over a fitted wool dress to create an unexpected take on the suit. Complementary shades of camel and brown plus almost-matching hemlines are what makes it feel "suit-y." Pointy-toed pumps inject a wink of sex appeal.

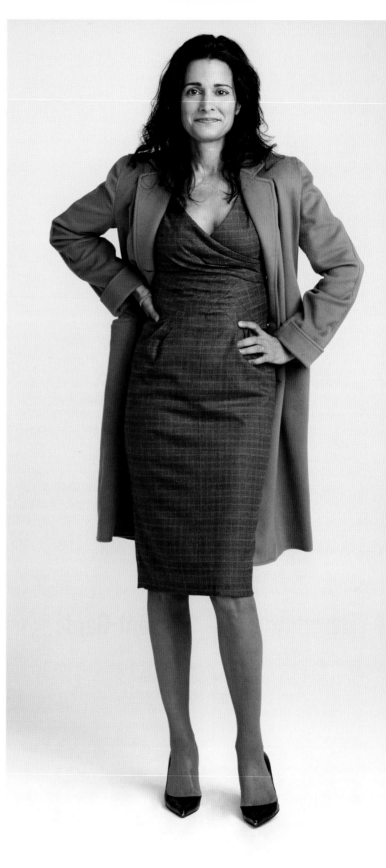

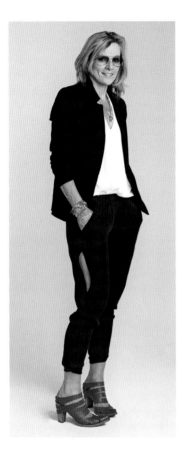

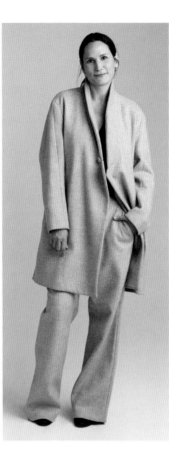

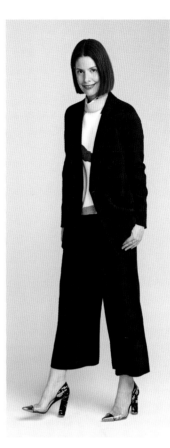

Case No. 2:
Downtown

Although Daryl is known for her rock-star styling, she still wears a suit on occasion—her own version, that is. While the jacket is classically tailored, Daryl added a side zipper to the pant leg, which can be left open or closed. Her tee (versus a conventional shirt) and cool pointy-toed clogs combine to form a dressed-down, creative office/work look.

Case No. 3:
Avant-Garde

It takes a certain kind of confidence to pull off April's oversize gray flannel pieces, from her Alasdair label. If you're not comfortable sporting big-on-big, swap the larger jacket for a fitted one or juxtapose an oversize coat with a slim pant; even a single outsize piece is interesting and cool.

Case No. 4:
Funky

Christene's vintage suit is appropriate for serious workdays or important events. But the daring choice of super-cropped wide-leg pants and an oversize jacket results in a more intriguing silhouette. Her suit is 1980s Armani; for a similar look, scour eBay, and then update your find with tailoring tweaks.

Getting the Most Out of Your Wardrobe

Turn One Look into Many

Most of your clothes are more versatile than you ever imagined. A single top and bottom can be split up to make so many outfits for different moods. Just look at Pascale's seemingly single-use all-red ensemble. It's perfect as is, but she can easily change its personality by adding and subtracting pieces.

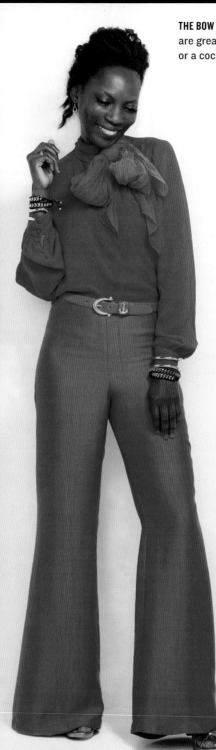

THE BOW BLOUSE AND TROUSERS are great on their own for work or a cocktail party.

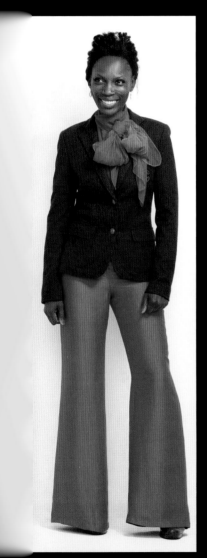

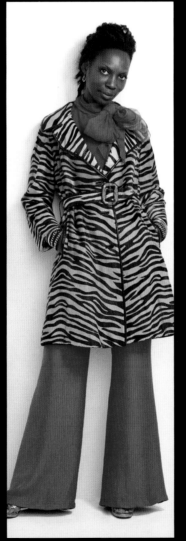

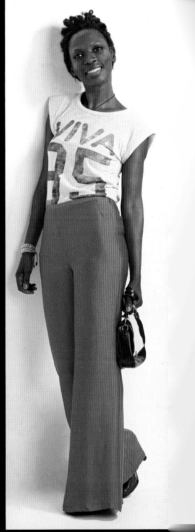

A TAILORED SCHOOLBOY BLAZER gives the look a more buttoned-up vibe.

A FUN ANIMAL-PRINT COAT dresses it up for a night out.

A CASUAL TEE replaces the blouse for a cooler, more playful attitude.

Q&A with Brooke Williams, Lifestyle Blogger

Name some fashion rules you live by.

Always be comfortable. Because you can't really be yourself if you are in pain or constantly tugging at a hemline. Never wear one designer/brand head to toe. Because you should be the author of your own look as opposed to a clothing brand, no matter how good it is. Don't show your stomach, except at the beach. Because let's be honest, at my age, nobody wants to see my stomach. When in doubt, lipstick, big sunglasses, and some good kicks will get you through almost any situation. Never forget that all rules are meant to be broken every once in a while.

Who are your favorite designers?

Maria Cornejo because her clothes are timeless and superintelligent and make me feel like a princess and a superhero at the same time. Tess Giberson because her clothes are a perfect combination of crafty hippie and gothic punk. Mona Kowalska (of A Détacher) because her clothes are weird and textural and otherworldly while still as familiar as a favorite hand-me-down from my mother. And on a more classic note, I love what Phoebe Philo is doing at Céline—the pieces are simultaneously austere and luxurious and look a bit like they come from an outer-space version

of the 1920s. Oh, and also vintage Dior and YSL, especially from the '50s and '60s, because they wrote the book, so to speak.

Go-to weekend outfit?

Since I work for myself, my weekends and weekdays are fairly interchangeable, though my weekends tend to be spent with my husband and daughter. If we're spending active time outdoors, I'm in jeans, a T-shirt, and sneakers. If we're out and about in the city, I'm more likely to be wearing a skirt or a dress. But I'm probably still wearing my kicks. I always carry a big bag, either from MZ Wallace or Mayle, full of snacks, a change of clothes for my daughter, water, a camera, etc.

Foolproof work outfit?

A pantsuit is my favorite thing to wear when I'm shooting. Plenty of pockets, supercomfortable, automatic polish. And that same oversize bag.

What did you used to wear all the time that you wouldn't dream of wearing now?

In college I wore hair extensions that I tied into a long ponytail because I wanted to look like Sade. I have no idea what I was thinking.

What is your favorite body part to emphasize?

I'd have to say my legs . . . I wear lots of short skirts.

Is there anything you do that breaks conventional fashion rules?

I mix patterns and wear all sorts of shades of the same color at once, I

don't shy away from combining brown and navy, and I happily wear white all winter long. But I don't think any of these "rules" really apply at this point, do they?

Do you have any fashion pet peeves?

People who are obsessed with labels and status drive me crazy. Fashion is fun and can be a vital form of self-expression, but it's not curing cancer or reversing global warming. It's so important to keep things in perspective. That said, developing your own personal style and feeling free to express your personality through the way you present yourself is an integral part of what makes the world such an interesting place to be.

Do you have any family beauty secrets that have been passed down or have stuck with you?

My mother taught me the importance of getting enough sleep (the answer to 90 percent of all problems!) and of wearing sunscreen. She also taught us (my sister and me) to apply body oil right before we get out of the shower because it locks in the extra moisture from the water. We used baby oil back in the day, but I've graduated to coconut oil. My father taught me the importance of drinking enough water—he starts every day with two glasses before he does anything.

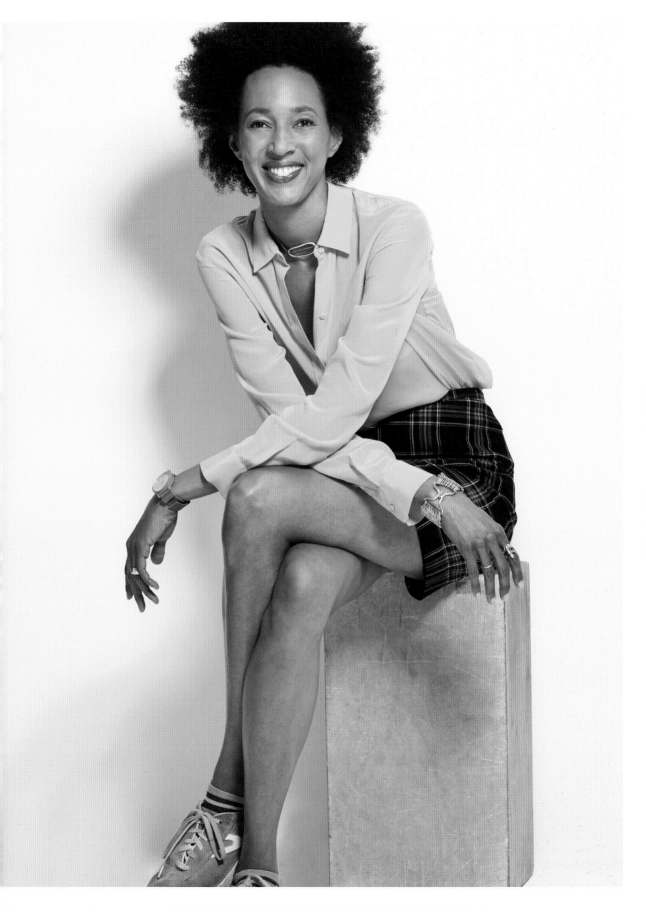

BLACK LEATHER IS NOT JUST FOR ROCKERS

When Clara Gaymard of GE France was photographed heading to a meeting with French president François Hollande in a motorcycle jacket a few years ago, women worldwide went leather-jacket crazy. It looked so great over Gaymard's somewhat conservative dress that even a super-corporate lawyer friend of mine hopped online to snap one up.

The appeal of rock 'n' roll dressing is undeniable. Who doesn't secretly wish she were a rock star (well, maybe just on the weekends)? Wearing clothes that evoke a mere whiff of rocker chic can make us feel cool and irreverent—even if it just means throwing on a pair of harness boots when running out for milk. As demonstrated by Gaymard, the biker jacket is becoming more acceptable no matter how conservative you are—or what age.

You might be surprised at how well leather can fit into many other style categories, from boho chic to classic Americana. Pair a leather skirt with a crisp white shirt and simple heels, and voilà: a European-inflected workday look. Style cropped leather pants with a cozy sweater and ankle boots or sweet loafers for elevated weekend wear.

Leather Staples for Everyone's Style

"Leather leggings are a twenty-first-century addition to the wardrobe of classics that will never go out of style. Only jeans can come close in comparison."

—Daryl Kerrigan

Case No. I:
Leather Leggings—
the New Jeans

Something as specific as a pair of black leather leggings can seem impractically one-note, but in fact, they're as versatile as a pair of jeans. This is the philosophy behind Daryl K leather and suede leggings. She makes some of the best, in all colors (see for yourself at darylk. com), and argues that every woman should own at least one pair. Here, the iconic designer proves her point by rocking them in her signature tough-girl style alongside Jennifer's more classic ensemble.

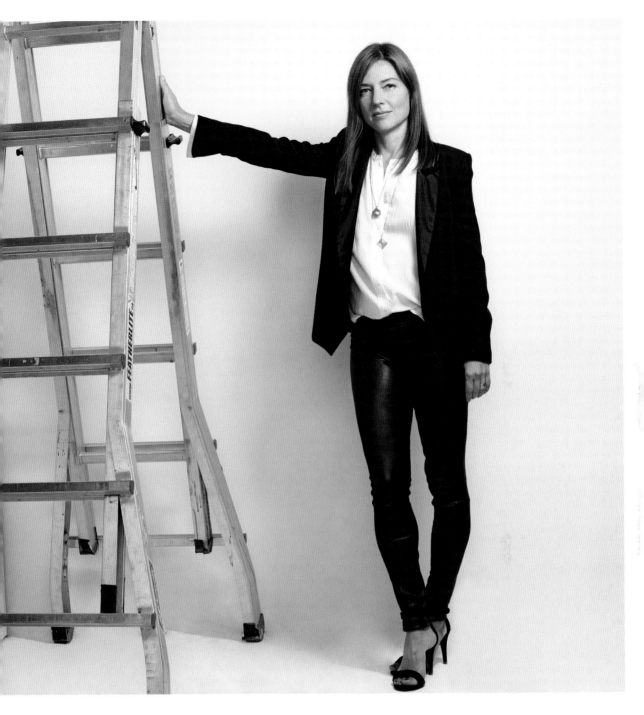

"There was a time when I was unsure I could pull off leather leggings, but now they're a staple in my wardrobe: I can't imagine life without them. I wear them with an oversize sweater and flat boots for day, heels and a tuxedo jacket at night."

—Jennifer Alfano

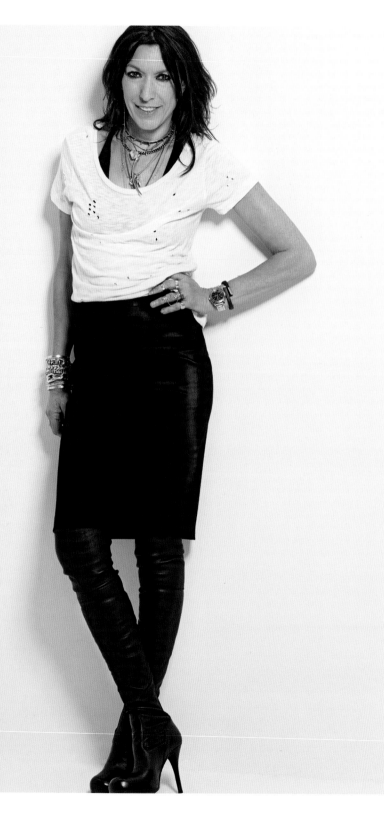

Case No. 2: Leather Pencil Skirt—an Unexpected Mainstay

Exhibit A: Mimi, who feels most at home in rock-star pieces like shaggy jackets and fierce black heels. Exhibit B: Susan, who is always classically dressed. Both love leather and consider pencil skirts everyday wardrobe staples. The point of difference here is in the styling.

ROCK 'N' ROLL. If you have the guts, go all-out with leather-on-leather like Mimi does. A tucked-in tee and a plain leather skirt take on a rock 'n' roll vibe when she adds sexy-tough thigh-high black leather boots—which continue the theme and lengthen her body.

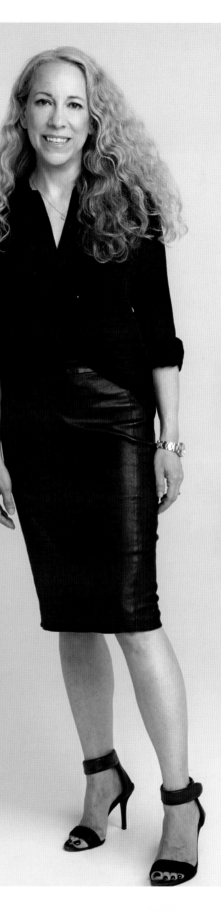

A SOFTER LOOK. Mimi rocks her leather hard, but that doesn't mean you have to. To make a leather pencil skirt more polished and less tough, follow Susan's lead and pair it with a feminine black (or cream) silk button-down and polished heels or strappy sandals. The look is office appropriate yet still sexy. Let the skirt be the star and keep everything else classic.

Case No. 3: Leather Miniskirt— Surprisingly Wearable

The very thought of a leather miniskirt probably sends shudders down your spine. But it's much easier to pull off than you'd imagine. Bear in mind that "mini" needn't mean crotch-grazing. A few inches above the knee is plenty short enough.

CITY SLICKER. The same rules apply for minis as they do for all other leather pieces: remember the "keep the leather the star" rule and all else will fall into place. Here, Karen pairs her miniskirt with a nice silk button-down and refined yet edgy high heels. Bare legs telegraph "urban chic" when the weather allows. (Crazy but true: all top magazine editors and stylists go bare-legged even in winter.)

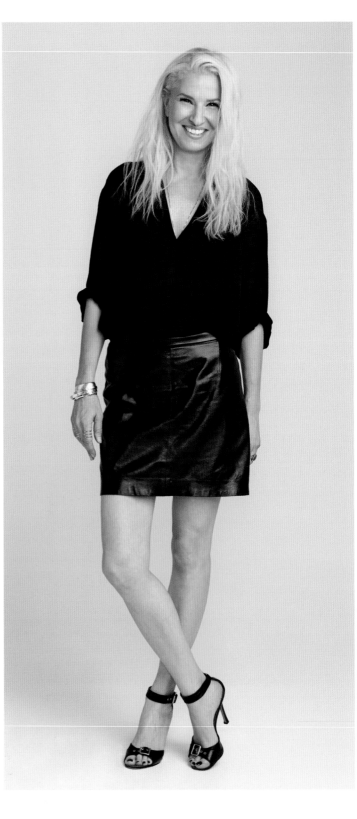

PUNKY. Vintage leather can be a great score. You just have to know how to make it look modern, not retro. Christina is all about mixing cool vintage of all kinds, which in this case helps temper the potential too-sexiness of a short leather skirt. She strategically dresses around the piece to make it look more "schoolgirl street" with black tights and a vintage camo jacket (which, worn with jeans, would read more tomboy).

The Skirt Has Two Faces

A seemingly prim accordion-pleated Prada skirt is utterly versatile in leather—as demonstrated by Lisa and Karen, who both showed up to the shoot with theirs. The to-the-knee length and unexpected material make the classically cut piece more all-purpose. Fancify it with a party jacket or a simple, thin cashmere sweater, and keep accompanying pieces pretty neutral.

SUPER CLASSIC. Lisa shows how leather can look European-luxe—just how Prada intended it. Her simple streamlined black cashmere sweater offsets the fullness of the skirt, while her '40s-style high-heeled sandals are feminine and understatedly sexy.

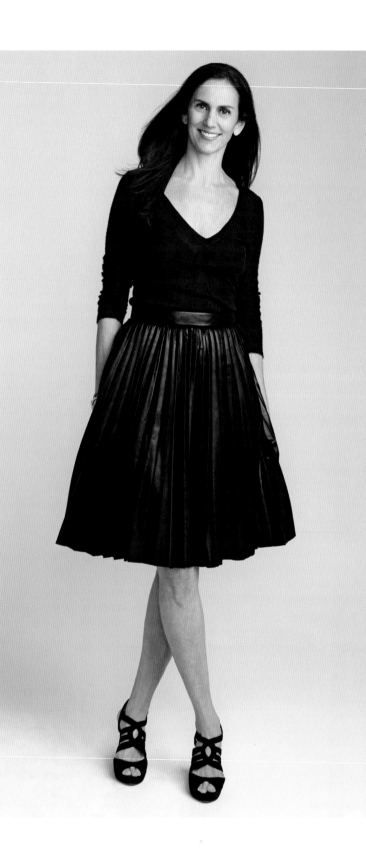

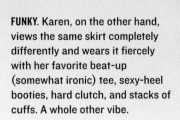

FUNKY. Karen, on the other hand, views the same skirt completely differently and wears it fiercely with her favorite beat-up (somewhat ironic) tee, sexy-heel booties, hard clutch, and stacks of cuffs. A whole other vibe.

Top It Off with Leather

Use leather as a wild card to bestow edge on an otherwise girlie (or too-classic) outfit. Tossing a leather vest or jacket over your most straightforward pairing brings it to a more interesting place. Leather outerwear is especially versatile since you can always remove it once indoors. And by adding a soft knit or silk scarf, you automatically soften the vibe.

AN UNEXPECTED TOPPER. Sometimes a simple, pretty dress is just begging for a little bad-boy action. I love the mix of hard and soft, heavy and light. Case in point: Kim's brightly hued, flowing silk dress, which turns casual-cool when she tops it with a tough biker jacket. Clunky black ankle boots add weight that nicely balances everything.

EDGY FEMININITY. Tina's favorite bohemian dress skews toward urban girlie, but she likes to feel a little edgy once in a while. A casual motorcycle vest over all of those frothy flowers toughens the look, as do the booties.

Leather Pants: More Versatile Than You'd Think

But alas, all are not created equal. Some leather pants are more classic, others more stage-worthy. And of course the vibe changes depending on what you've got on top. This is a great opportunity to breathe new life into your most basic pieces. Here are some options.

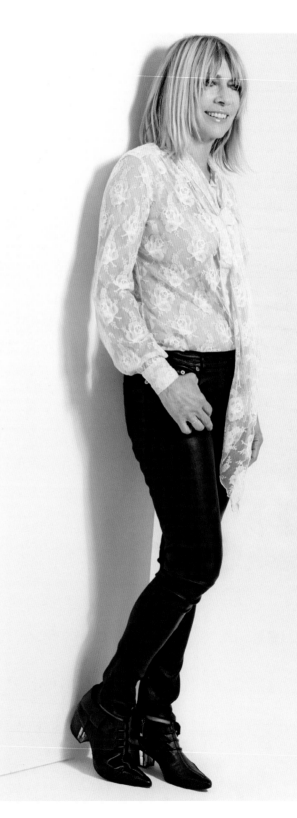

SOFTER ROCK. For a hard-edged yet feminine look, pair classic five-pocket (i.e., jeans-style) leather pants with a lacy or plain silk bow blouse. Kim's inspired result: one part Jimi Hendrix, one part French film star.

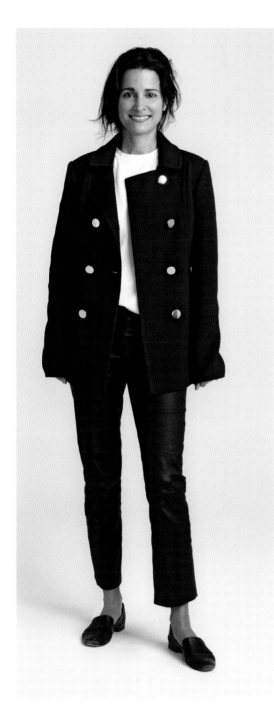

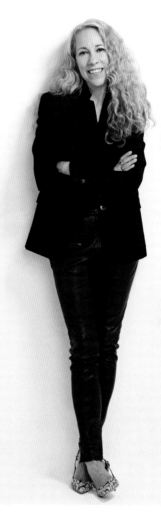

FIT TIP: Leather pants should be buttery (otherwise they could feel too masculine or biker-chick or add extra bulk), and should fit like your favorite pair of skinny jeans: comfy-snug through the seat, slim on the leg. Buy them as tight as you can stand, since they'll stretch and mold to your body. (This dictum is especially true with leggings.) Also make sure they're lined at least to just above the shin (pants, not leggings, which have more stretch), which will keep them from bagging out at the knee.

SPORTY-CLASSIC. Anna favors her leathers slightly cropped for a sweeter silhouette. She wears them like any other trousers: with a white tee, a shrunken peacoat, and loafers. The look is Euro-preppy, but much less so than if the pants were wool.

POLISHED. Susan can totally wear her leathers to meetings if she pairs them with a black silk blouse, a tailored jacket, and python sling backs—all of which keep everything polished and feminine.

ANATOMY OF

The Classic Biker Jacket

If you're going to go for just one amazing leather piece, make it the grandfather of them all: the classic motorcycle jacket. The right one will never look dated. Just stick with old-school detailing for a piece you'll love wearing with everything—and forever. Here's what to look for.

A SNAP-DOWN COLLAR (that you will leave unsnapped).

JUST ENOUGH ZIPPERAGE. The classic jacket has four zippers (the main one plus three zippered pockets).

A ZIPPERED SLEEVE to wear open or closed.

EPAULETS—they're classic, but you can go without if you want something more refined.

A TINY POCKET ON THE BOTTOM SIDE (originally designed for coins).

A SELF BELT, meant to be worn open when the jacket is open. (I also like this no-belt version.)

SAINT LAURENT
PARIS

Q&A with Daryl Kerrigan, Fashion Designer

What was your first fashion splurge and why?

A pair of Barbara Hulanicki (Biba) shoes that I bought in Dublin when I was in high school. They were part gladiator sandals, part winklepicker flats that laced up the ankle. I was one of the few who knew who Barbara was because my mom had bought cool stuff at her store in London. I see similar shoes around today.

Who are your style icons?

They change through the years. In my club-kid days it was comic book superheroines, and later iconic male rock stars like David Bowie and Michael Jackson or movie stars like Clint Eastwood. But generally I have more style moods and looks that inspire me rather than actual style icons.

Name some fashion rules you live by.

I don't know if I have any "rules"—I like breaking them! But I must be true to my personal style and also express my current style mood, which could be influenced by anything from my environment or music to the weather. Minimalism is always important. I don't like to break up the body too much with a lot of prints and colors, and I've always got to feel free to move and be unconstricted. Too much fashion isn't my style either.

Foolproof work outfit?

Leather leggings, silk shirt, jacket.

Foolproof evening or party look?

It changes, but layers are important for different times of the evening—early, dinner, dancing. . . .

What are your favorite accessories?

Gold and silver jewelry, and diamonds! I keep the same pieces on for a year or more, then switch to something new.

Is there anything you do that breaks conventional fashion rules?

Definitely. I always have been a rule breaker, but now that's a trend and I don't like being trendy.

Do you only have expensive designer clothing or do you mix?

I don't care what the label is as long as I love the quality and design of the piece.

Is there anything you've owned and worn for more than fifteen years?

A black leather Daryl K jacket.

Do you have any family beauty secrets that have been passed down or have stuck with you?

Healthy food, some exercise every day, water with lemon juice.

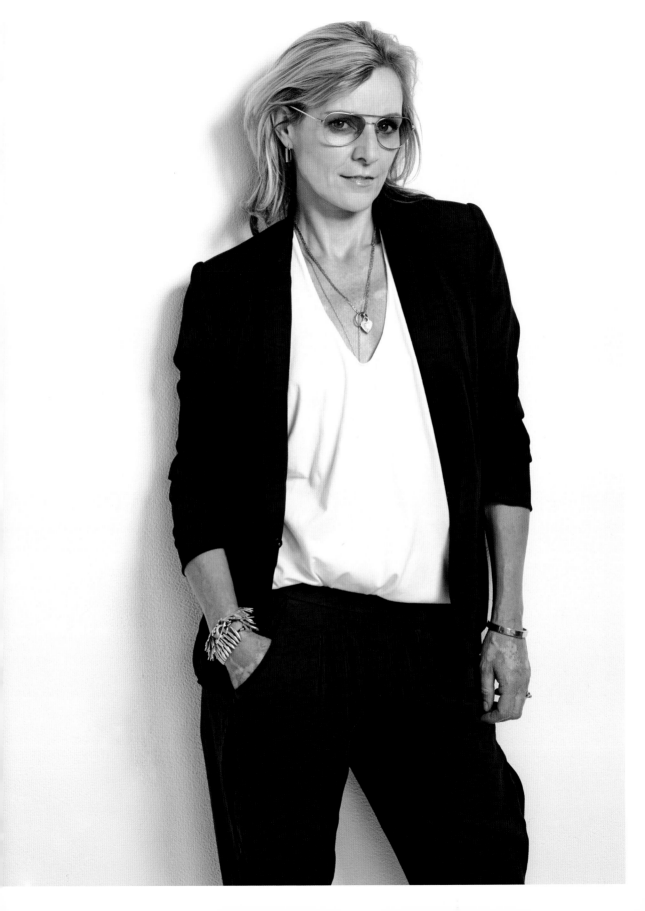

DRESSING DOESN'T HAVE TO SEND YOU INTO A TIZZY

My sister, Dana, and I recently attended a family wedding at Hampton Court, a palace just outside London. The dreaded words "black tie" on the invite sent us over the edge. What does the term even mean these days? Is a floor-length gown mandatory? Everything became a source of stress, from what hairstyle was suitable to what jewelry would be deemed adequately formal.

To calm myself, I envisioned women like Maria Cornejo and April Johnson, who would undoubtedly wear some cool, slouchy design from their own label. They'd just be . . . themselves.

I am so *not* a gown person, and while Dana looks better in a flowing formal number than I do, she really isn't either. So for the rehearsal dinner I dared to wear a loose lamé pantsuit (from April's Alasdair line, in fact), and I felt much more *me*— and much more comfortable—than I would have in the requisite fancy cocktail dress. And for the wedding itself, I scored a long '70s vintage tiered chiffon number that could pass for 1930s Chanel. Dana went for an elegant yet plain black floor-length dress with a slight train.

The best part of the evening? That everyone interpreted black tie differently—and yet still looked totally appropriate. Some women wore tight dresses; others donned drapey ones. My favorite was a long, simple slip dress in burgundy silk worn by a woman with messy hair piled atop her head and super-big, slightly bohemian beaded earrings. When I asked who made it, she replied, "Nili Lotan—it's really just a beach dress." Truly chic women, those with inimitable personal style, do their own thing for *every* occasion—no matter how fancy.

Day-to-Night Cocktails

Who has time to run home after work to change out of her office attire and into dress-up clothes? Better to spend the entire day in an outfit that swings both ways. Wearing something over-the-top with a casual piece will take the edge off both extremes—and create an outfit that looks appropriate almost anywhere. Try deflating the seriousness of formalwear by pairing a froufrou frock with an everyday shoe, for instance.

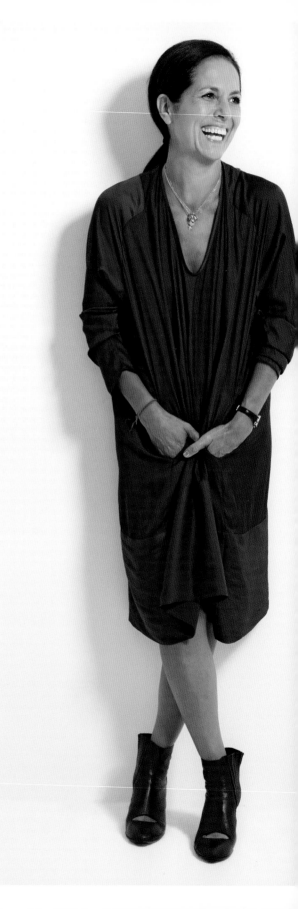

DRESSED-UP TEE. Maria's T-shirt-y dress can easily play the chameleon: completely casual when worn with flip-flops and a suntan, or party-pretty with heels and statement-making jewelry. What makes this particular dress work for more formal occasions is its fluidness: silky and drapey, it's body skimming but not clingy.

DRAMATIC. April's austere wool dress looks serious by day and, courtesy of its angular drape and intriguing origami-esque folds, surprisingly festive at night. Note the higher neckline, which counterintuitively amplifies the drama. Shoe booties are avant-garde glamorous yet still comfortable after a 9-to-5 shift.

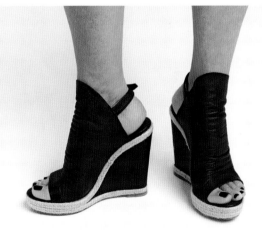

TIP: Don't neglect your toes! Choose a polish that complements the *attitude* of your outfit. Dark tones like black and burgundy are the epitome of cool glamour, like this elegant shade on Jeanine. But I also love a sheer toe: Jin Soon's Tulle is one of my favorites.

The Coy Factor

Many women make the mistake of revealing every imaginable body part, thinking that's how to look sexy after sundown. Not so. Be strategic and a little withholding. Think understated— not overexposed.

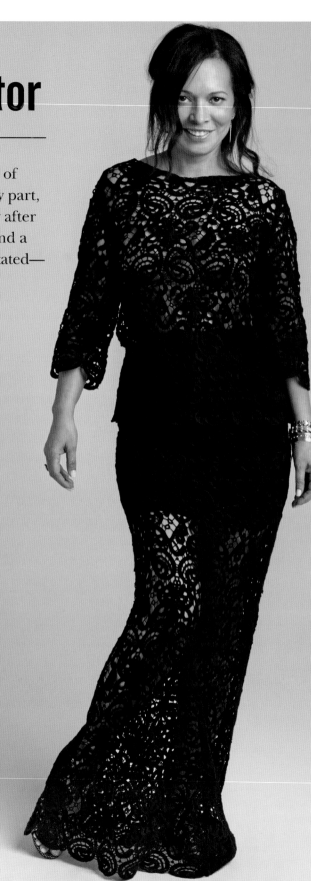

THE PEEKABOO EFFECT. Miguelina's outfit is sexy but not obviously so. Rather than flaunt the usual cleavage or too much leg, she covers up with a sheer lace gown and a strategic slip—creating a sort of layer-cake effect—that lets her silhouette peek through the fabric. Yet she's completely sheathed except for her wrists, which are set off by a bracelet-length sleeve. Adornments are kept to the bare minimum; a dress this decorated is jewelry in itself.

THE BARE-ARM EFFECT. Kim's sheer-top dress mimics a strapless bustier, but the gauzy lace covers like a long-sleeved dress (while adding interest). Much sultrier and chicer—not to mention more forgiving—than bare skin would be. It's like showing off your arms, but through a Photoshop filter. The short dress/long sleeve combo is always a winner.

A Little Boho Goes a Long, Long Way

Lest you think you need some serious, stuffy gown for a fancy affair, consider these two takes on hippie chic. Both are unconventional yet party-ready. To pull off the look, select pieces that are perfectly tailored, and style them with clean-lined modern accents.

HIPPIE CHIC. While Anne wouldn't wear this folkloric dress to a buttoned-up bash, spot-on tailoring and perfect proportions make the flea-market find completely evening appropriate. The fit is snug in the shoulders, the bracelet-length sleeves show off a sliver of wrist, and the skirt isn't so long that it covers her shoes; in this case, floor length would be *less* dressy (and more muumuu-ish). Styling trick: modern ankle-tie shoes keep it from veering costumey.

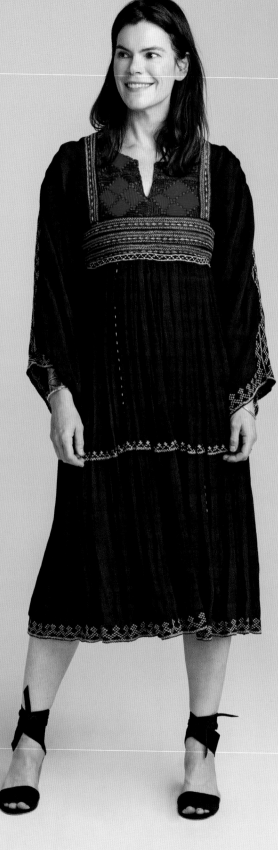

FOR ALL-OUT DRAMA, THINK BIG. (AND COMFY!) Janis forgoes the usual tailored gown, opting instead for a long and voluminous wing-sleeved chiffon number that's one step away from a beach caftan. Supremely chic—yet secretly cozy. What keeps such a billowing design from screaming "bikini cover-up!" is her simple blown-out hair, the bare neckline, and perfectly chosen accessories. Because her amazing cuffs are chunky and substantial, they make a powerful statement.

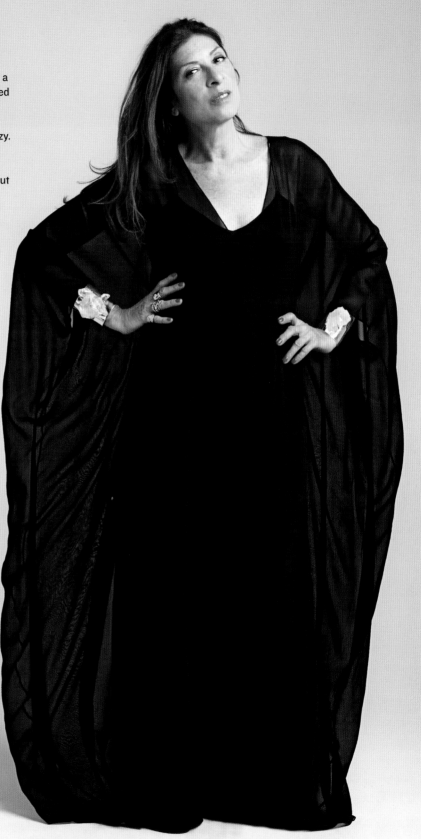

Little Black Dress Alternatives

Yes, black is foolproof and failsafe, but if you're into standing out, go in the opposite direction. Think outside the box: avoid anything over-the-top or obvious. Pore through your closet and dare to give non-dressy pieces a chance in the limelight.

LONG AND LIVELY. Susan's floor-sweeping patterned dress is surprisingly serious—swank enough even for a black-tie summertime bash. And yet worn with flip-flops, it's suitably casual for weekend wear or a Saturday afternoon get-together.

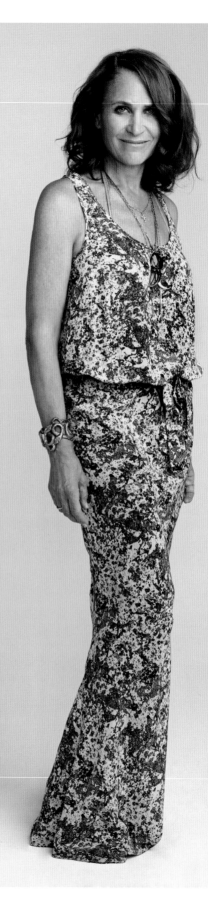

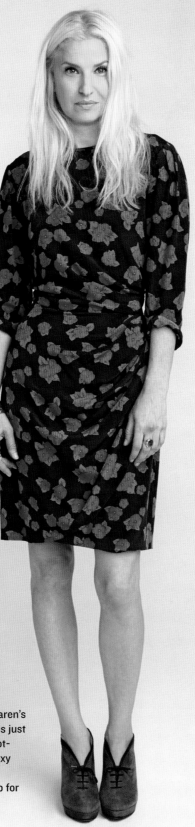

Fancify Your Everyday Attire with These Accessories

- **STATEMENT EARRINGS.** Dangly chandeliers always do the trick, adding just the right dose of femininity. They're an immediate signifier of fanciness, almost distracting attention from whatever else you're wearing.

- **A JUST-BIG-ENOUGH EVENING BAG.** It only needs to hold the essentials, so you can prioritize form over function. Opt for a super-sleek satin clutch, a delicate chain-strap shoulder bag, or a sparkly beaded drawstring pouch.

- **RIGHT-HEIGHT HEELS.** Just tall enough to look fabulous, but low enough that you can walk properly and comfortably (a height that's different for everyone). Choose a refined, elegant silhouette: a slightly curved or straight thin heel versus a chunky one.

- **EYES *OR* MOUTH—NEVER BOTH.** Go for smoky eye makeup or a strong, not-too-glossy lipstick, but please stick with one.

FLOWERS ARE ALWAYS FESTIVE. Karen's vintage designer floral dress is just right for a cocktail party or not-too-buttoned-up wedding. Sexy booties lend edginess, while strappy heels would step it up for a more conservative event.

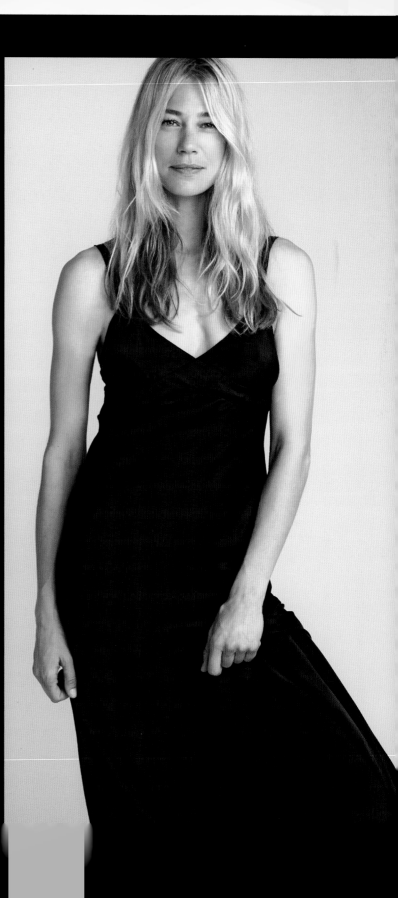

Getting the Most Out of Your Wardrobe

One Simple Silk Slip Can Be So Many Things!

Alone, the dress is a blank canvas. Pretty and simple on its own, but transformable into so many looks.

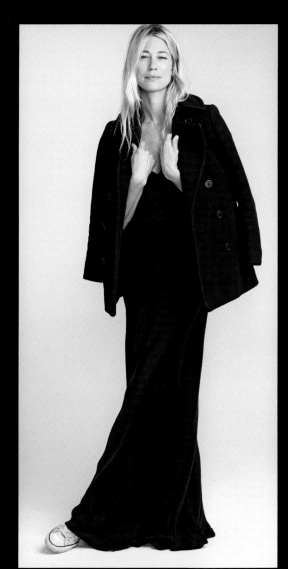

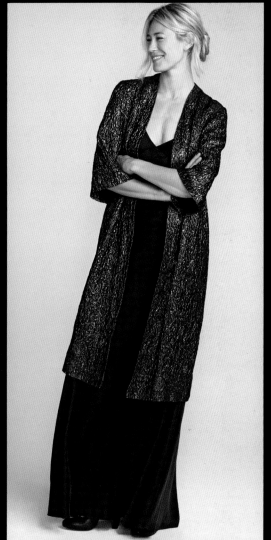

For day, Caroline wears it with her perfect military peacoat and Converse low-tops—a great outfit for spring or fall.

For a whole new mood, throw something fancier on top, like Caroline's cool vintage gold evening duster. She also pulls her hair back in a messy bun, and— boom!—she's ready for a party.

Q&A with Maria Cornejo, Fashion Designer

What was your first fashion splurge and why?

A Vivienne Westwood corset. I bought it in 1981 when I was in college. I wore it with men's pants. It was my first big purchase. She was (and is) so amazing.

What are the items in your closet that you've had the longest and will never throw out?

Because my family fled Chile, I didn't grow up with anything from my childhood, so I keep everything. I have every collection I've ever done in the basement of my home. I'll never throw out the first collection I did in college.

Name some fashion rules you live by.

Don't try to be something other than yourself, be comfortable, rejoice in your good points, less is more, color is more, one piece works best.

Foolproof work outfit?

A jumpsuit.

What is your favorite body part to emphasize?

My legs. It makes me feel taller and I like to wear pants and jumpsuits because they make me look longer.

Any good styling tricks? Belting, layering, rolling, cropping?

I love layering and belting with big volume.

Any signature beauty or hair thing you do?

I always pull back my hair, and I wear red lipstick when I go out, but otherwise I'm pretty natural.

Any length and fit rules you do or don't follow?

No pants or skirts that hit mid-calf. I don't think it's flattering.

Do you have any fashion pet peeves?

Handbag dogs, the really tiny ones.

Is there anything you've owned and worn for more than fifteen years?

A navy fireman jacket from Paris.

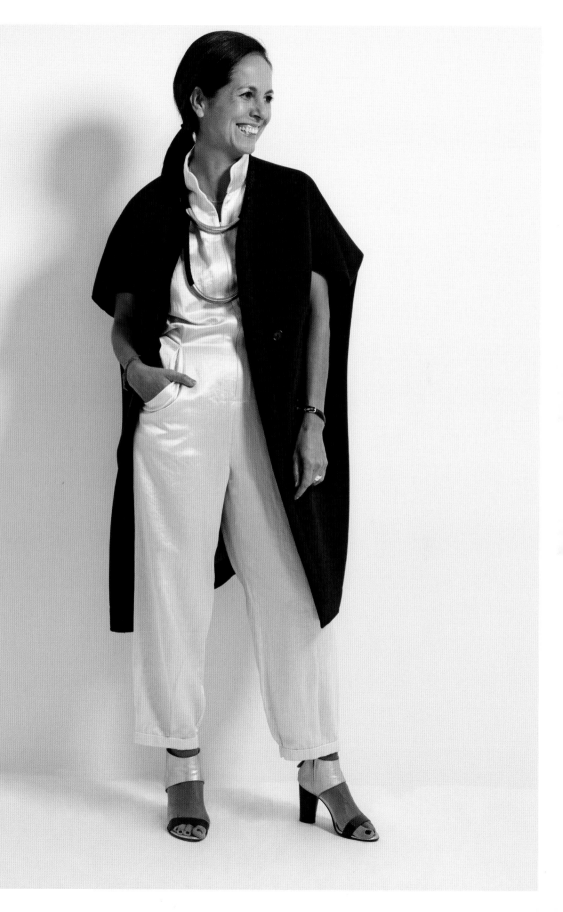

YOU CAN'T HAVE STYLE WITHOUT ACCESSORIES

The easiest way to change a look has nothing to do with the pieces themselves, but with the extra goodies you add to them. It's actually kind of crazy how jewelry, scarves, and even hats can make an outfit say something completely different than what it said a minute before. For example, you can take a plain, minimalist black dress and wear it as is for an unfussy vibe, or add an ethnic bib necklace—and you suddenly exude artsiness. Lose the bib and tie on a bright scarf and you become that much more interesting (plus, bright colors add flush to the cheeks). Like I said, accessories make the woman.

The Power of Accessories

The easiest way to change a look is not to reconsider the pieces of clothing you've put together but to add fun jewelry or some other detail to the outfit. For instance, a pair of plain jeans and a white tee are pretty perfect on their own—but with the right additions, you can realize abundant looks, from glam to classic. Here are some examples.

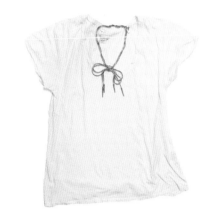

An interesting designer bow necklace turns the tee into an elegant top.

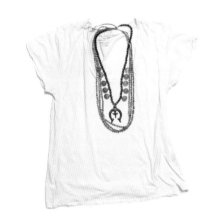

A mix of vintage Native American turquoise and silver lends ethnic chic.

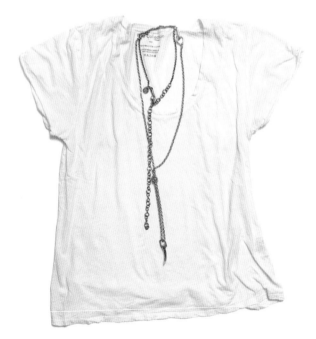

Layered heavy gold chains add a dose of sexy glamour.

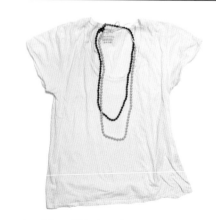

A pairing of black and white pearls creates a French lady effect.

Other Ways to Reinvent a White Tee

Jewelry and other accessories are great to have on hand to turn your basic tees into an outfit that tells a real story.

- **ADD TONS OF PEARLS**, a fancy watch, ballet flats, and a petite quilted chain-strap bag and you're a hip Parisian—à la French icon Inès de la Fressange.

- **PILE ON SILVER BANGLES**, oversize hoops (not too wiry), a chunky man's watch, and classic leather jodhpur boots for a cool country/urban look.

- **WEAR WITH OVERSIZE CHANDELIER DROP EARRINGS** and pointy-toed stilettos and you're party ready.

- **OR FORGO JEWELRY ALTOGETHER** and twist a little Hermès foulard or classic cotton bandana around your neck for a sweet French or classic Americana look.

Chic rock 'n' roller Mimi really believes more is more. She piles on a whole tangle of her favorite heavy silver chains and edgy pendants that help to create her signature look.

Shoes Can Make or Break an Outfit

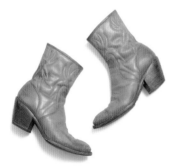

Behold my all-time favorite cowboy boots with the narrow zip-up ankle. Mine are old Chloé, but you can take a real pair to your shoe guy and have him put in a zipper to create a similar pair.

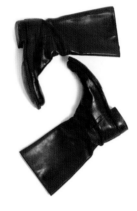

You can't go wrong with classic brown leather rancher boots like Lisa's. Perfect under or over jeans or with midi skirts.

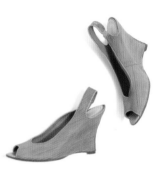

April's walkable wedge sandals give a '70s girlie appeal to all of her avant-garde pieces.

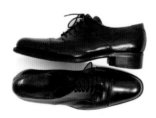

Linda's great oxfords lend a little cool masculinity to dresses, trousers, and jeans.

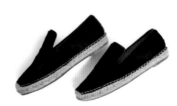

A pair of simple classic flat espadrilles like Bibi's are a great summer staple.

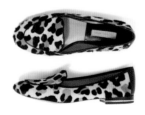

Anna's cute leopard loafers are for days when she wants a little more oomph.

Shoes are my weakness; most likely, the same goes for you. Why? Because they set the tone by establishing the "language" of your outfit. Take a simple, elemental pairing: a black A-line skirt and a V-neck cashmere sweater. Slide on your favorite broken-in Arizona Birkenstocks for a laid-back, slightly edgy weekend look. Don men's-style brogues and you're an androgynous-chic Manhattanite. Try a stacked-heel knee-high boot instead, and the effect is sexy '70s. Three entirely different looks—without changing a single article of clothing.

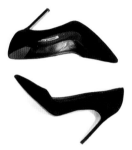

The right black pumps like Jennifer's (just pointy enough, with a nice dip near the toe and a fierce heel) can turn anyone into a *French Vogue* editor.

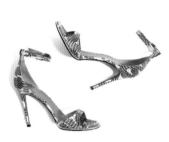

Everyone needs at least one standout pair of sexy streamlined high-heeled sandals like Anamaria's to turn any outfit into an evening one.

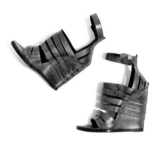

Karen's übersexy wedges turn her skinny jeans into something much more glamorous.

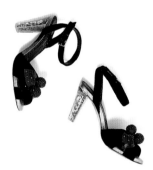

Janis's kooky Carmen Miranda heels add humor to even the most austere black dress.

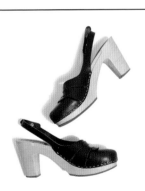

A more grown-up, polished version of the beloved clog from Caroline's closet.

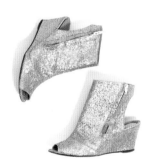

Kim's sparkly silver shoes are a little-girl princess fantasy with a punk-rock twist.

What Your Bag Says About You

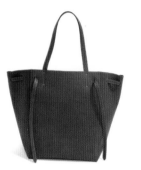

Jennifer's clean no-hardware tote in a rich brown screams, "I am chic and understated!"

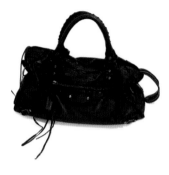

Molly's Balenciaga City bag says, "I'm a bit boho-edgy but still appreciate the classics."

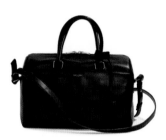

Susan Kaufman's Saint Laurent Speedy has a timeless European "lady" shape.

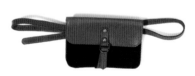

A sleek fanny pack like Gayle's holds essentials and leaves your hands free—wear with a tote or alone.

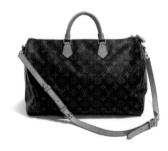

A Louis Vuitton Speedy (size 40) is my go-to carry-on and work bag. It elevates even my most casual outfits.

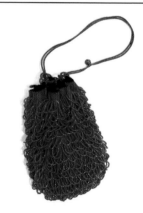

Anne's sweet little beaded evening bag is vintage boho glam.

The bag you choose to carry is almost as impactful as your shoes. I have more bags than I care to admit—one for every mood: fringed hippie ones, structured lady satchels, utilitarian denim totes . . . the list goes on. Although, unlike your shoes, you usually stash away your bag once you arrive at your destination, this essential accessory still plays a major role in your overall look. Here are some optimal choices, each of which telegraphs an entirely different vibe.

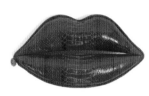

Janis's evening bag is just pure sexy fun.

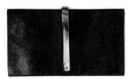

Maria's sophisticated black clutch reads, "I'm cool and unfussy."

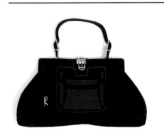

Susan Kaufman's vintage trompe l'oeil Roberta di Camerino shows a sense of style and a great sense of humor.

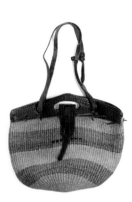

Scosha's African sisal carryall is the antifashion bohemian choice.

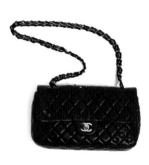

Jeanine's Chanel Ladybug bag is classic with a funny twist that says, "I love luxury, but I don't take myself too seriously!"

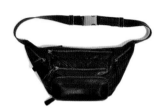

A fanny pack from Daryl Kerrigan's collection conveys a utilitarian cool with a bit of '80s irony.

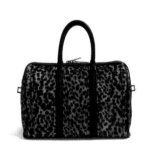

A leopard version of my Speedy from Tina is both fun and chic.

The Perfect Jewelry Box

What Everyone Should Own

- **GOLD BANGLES.** The awesome sound of clanking and the richness of the gold elevate anything else you're wearing. Costume works too!

- **DIAMOND STUDS.** Real or fake, they add just enough sparkle and can make you feel polished even when you're dressed down. Check out Jennifer Miller and Erwin Pearl for some of the many great fake ones out there.

- **WHITE PEARL STUDS.** They aren't for everyone, but when they're right, they're *right*. I especially love them on dark-skinned and dark-haired women.

- **BLACK PEARLS.** These look cool on everyone.

- **BIG GOLD HOOPS.** Sexy and face-framing.

- **BIG SILVER HOOPS.** Ditto, yet more casual.

Just as I'm obsessed with shoes and bags, I go bananas for all genres of jewelry. Over the years, I've accrued everything from antique rose-cut diamond rings to bold Native American turquoise cuffs. Collecting jewelry is not only fun but also a styling savior, pulling you out of a fashion rut (especially in the dead of winter, when you're feeling less than dynamic). And you don't have to spend a fortune on real gems or rare pieces—even a cool street find can add the needed excitement that turns a simple outfit into something more special.

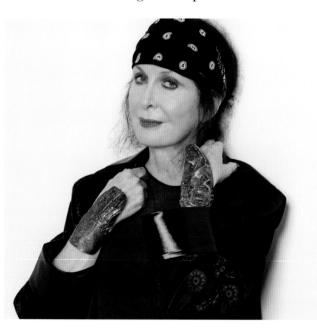

Linda usually leaves the fun up to her outfit and forgos most jewelry (aside from her stellar antique diamond ring). But for special occasions she does love the extra pizzazz she gets from her amazing structural cuffs.

Fun Pieces That Add Interest

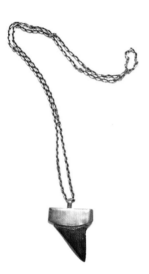

I love this oversize shark-tooth pendant and wear it when I want to feel a tad fierce.

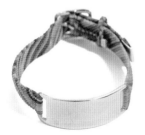

Scosha's unisex macramé ID bracelet is the perfect mix of classic and boho.

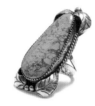

Sometimes all I need is my giant turquoise ring, which adds a bit of cool Americana drama to anything.

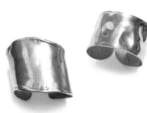

Bold modern cuffs in silver or gold create a little drama. Not for the meek, these are meant to be *seen*.

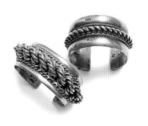

Ethnic cuffs—Native American, Afghani, Berber, and African—are divine and bring something very cool to a plain black crewneck or a classic button-down.

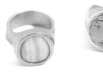

Scosha mixes rings from her own collection to create an interesting jewelry story.

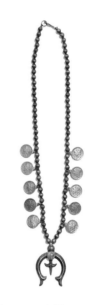

My silver squash blossom necklace is a true American classic that looks great over a simple black dress or white tee or under a menswear button-down.

TIP: Convert a regular strand of pearls into something much cooler—and a bit sexy—by having it restrung either with colored thread or in a different order than the usual graduated style, or both.

Throw On a Hat and Feel Instantly Cool

Hats change a look by adding attitude and drama. But they can be tricky to pull off without looking like you've tried too hard. If this concerns you, reserve them for days when the weather—rain, strong sun, freezing temperatures—merits wearing one so it's serving a purpose, too.

Tina is one of those people who can get away with effortless-seeming hat wearing. Her slightly crushed men's-style fedora dresses up her favorite jeans and sweater, making the ensemble more of a "look."

When Karen wants to create a little glam-rock story, she adds her cute felt hat.

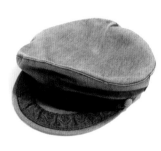

I love Christina's denim Greek fisherman cap. And the fact that it's beat-up and faded from the sun gives it all the more personality.

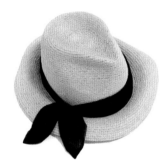

Kaela's straw hat is a bit girlier than your usual fedora, and the bow adds even more sweetness. A nice juxtaposition with ripped jeans and cool shoes (see page 42).

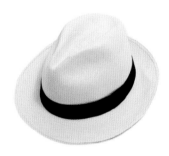

Miguelina's panama hat keeps the sun away and looks super vacation-y and mellow.

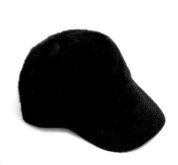

An angora "baseball" hat is Daryl's cold-weather go-to.

TIP: Most women look best when they leave a little hair peeking out of the hat to frame the face.

Nothing Changes an Outfit Quite Like a Scarf

Scarves add so much to a look. I have super-big bandanas that can wrap a few times around the neck, all kinds of cashmere versions—from wispy-light to winter-thick—long, skinny silk neck wraps to dress up a blouse or tee . . . this book isn't long enough to list them all. My must-have list of essentials includes all that's required to complete any look.

When you're pure rock 'n' roll like Mimi, a little color around the face helps break up all that black, as with her Sex Pistols scarf.

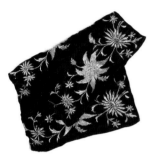

A beautiful embroidered shawl is what Susan Kaufman wears to add a little drama to an evening outfit.

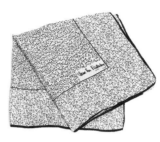

A sexy '70s silk scarf like Christina's adds instant vintage cool to a plain button-down or tee.

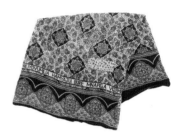

This is one of my favorites—it's actually an African sarong from the Ivory Coast, but I love to wear it as a scarf.

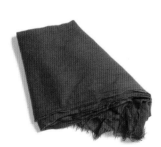

A pretty pashmina in a bright shade is perfect to buffer summer air-conditioning. Keep it stashed in your bag and wrap it around your shoulders as needed.

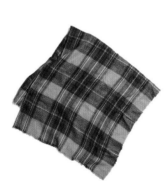

A giant, soft blanket scarf is all you need for super-cold days. It doesn't have to be fancy cashmere; I have a few amazing acrylic ones from Asos that cost about twenty-five dollars each—and that I always get complimented on. (Don't knock the synthetics: acrylic is incredibly soft!)

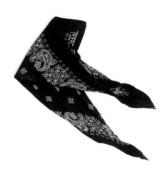

Classic blue, black, or red bandanas are great for the beach (on your neck or head), or to wear with a white tee or button-down or under an itchy turtleneck.

Q&A with Linda Dresner, Boutique Owner

What was your first fashion splurge and why?

A camel suit from Tiffeau & Busch. I was in my early twenties, a young mother and modeling . . . I felt sophisticated.

Describe your beauty routine, including products used.

My hair is curly, and I stopped blow-drying it when I went to Thailand with my future third husband. I was panicked—he had never seen my natural hair—but he said, "I love it." That was that. For my skin, I have been having laser treatments for about six years, and I use Neova products on the advice of my dermatologist.

How would you describe your style? How has it evolved over the years?

I wear what I want—a combination of old Comme des Garçons, Jean Muir, Yohji Yamamoto, and Martin Margiela and new pieces.

What are the items in your closet that you've had the longest and will never throw out?

These items can be twenty-plus years old . . . if I can button them, I wear them. Some things from Thea Porter and Zandra Rhodes are still in my closet; I'm hoping that my granddaughters will want to wear them—they are old enough and beautiful— but I'm still waiting for them to say yes.

Name some fashion rules you live by.

DO NOT LOOK LIKE YOU HAVE TRIED TOO HARD!

Go-to weekend outfit?

At home, baggy old jeans and a black long-sleeved crew neck cotton stretch T-shirt (ten dollars from Walmart) . . . and perfume and eye makeup. I cook on the weekends. Or some old Comme des Garçons long, loose dresses when we have company. Also flat sandals.

Foolproof work outfit?

A version of the above [jeans look]—without holes.

What did you used to wear all the time that you wouldn't dream of wearing now?

A girdle.

What is your favorite body part to emphasize?

I have good legs; they are the last to go, you know.

Is there anything you wear every single day?

A black Wolford cotton bodysuit, so in case I'm in an accident I won't be humiliated with the wrong underwear.

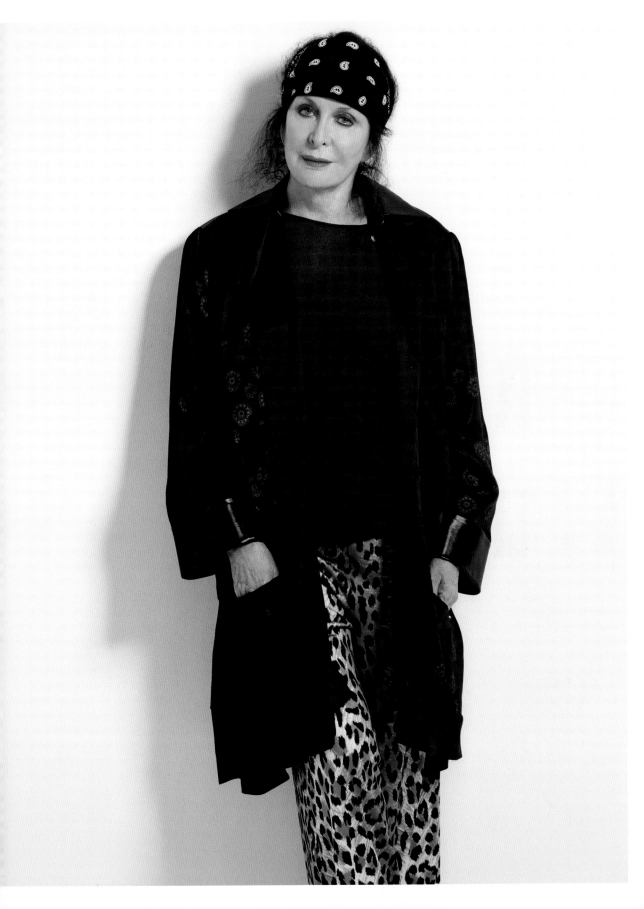

HAIR
(AND MAKEUP)
CAN BE
YOUR BIGGEST
FASHION
STATEMENT

Long or short? Hide or flaunt your gray? Highlights or single process? There are so many ways to express your individual style through what's growing on your head. When I was younger, I experimented with all sorts of looks: spiky rock 'n' roll Rod Stewart layers, super-short bangs cut into my hairline so they unfortunately resembled a nailbrush (really), a cute-yet-too-trendy asymmetric bob. But now I feel most comfortable just letting my hair *be*: wavy, long, and nice. (Although I do get the French-girl-bangs urge now and then.)

You can find good hair inspiration anywhere—in magazines, on the street, even on the movie screen—but heed this caveat: before you dash to the salon with that inspiration photo in hand, solicit a second opinion from a really good, really honest friend (the one who tells you when you have food in your teeth or when your jeans really aren't flattering). And then make sure the cut suits *your* face, *your* hair type, and *your* style—the hair has to look good on *you*. Be realistic: accept that your fine blond hair will never achieve the effect of that chic brunette's curly bob.

The secret to hair and makeup is to work with what you have. The goal is to look healthy and at your total, amazing best. Accentuate your favorite features—in the most natural way possible—and you're golden.

Long or Short?

So many women chop their hair off when they reach a certain age because they think they're supposed to. Hello: There's no legislature that dictates sensible hair after forty-five! If you have good, healthy hair, I see no reason to ever cut it (other than a trim now and then, of course). Keep it long if it works for your face shape and style. I've always admired women like Tricia Jones, co-founder of *i-D* magazine, and the actress Sonia Braga, who both have gorgeous long hair and would never snip it just to follow the "rules."

I happen to look better with long hair. That said, as soon as it grows to a certain length—several inches past my shoulders—I start feeling like an old hippie and chop it to just a few inches below my collarbone. Long or short or somewhere in between, just make sure your hair makes *you* feel good.

"I keep my hair long because it's really low maintenance. Or, rather, because I'm downright lazy. I do not have time to blow-dry, apply product to, or fuss with my hair. When I was growing up in Italy and Brooklyn, my grandmothers did the fussing. They would spray my hair with tea made from fresh chamomile and lemon to preserve the natural highlights (it worked). They also braided my hair and coated it with olive oil and jasmine flowers—way before those same ingredients were bottled and sold at Sephora."

—Laura Ferrara

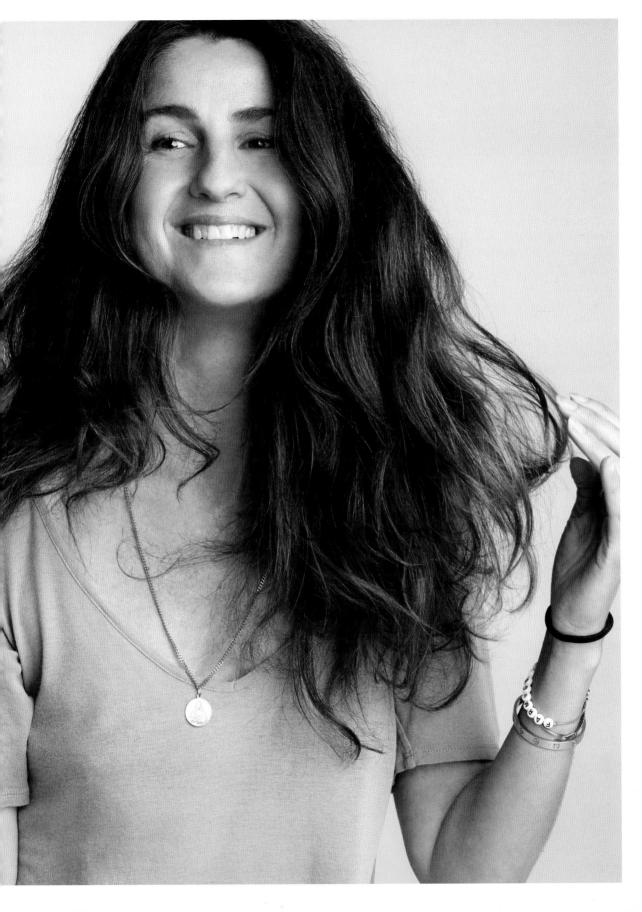

What Looks Great with Long Hair

- **MENSWEAR.** Pieces like oversize trousers create a nice masculine/feminine juxtaposition.

- **BUTTON-DOWNS.** Fresh and equestrian—think classic Ralph Lauren.

- **SHORT-SLEEVED OR SLEEVELESS T-SHIRTS.** Long hair looks great cascading over bare arms.

- **LEATHER JACKETS.** Lengthy locks keep them from looking too manly.

- **SKINNY JEANS.** Could there be a sexier combo?

- **TOMBOY SNEAKERS LIKE CONVERSE.** Again, it's all about the contrast.

- **PINSTRIPES.** Another take on the menswear-meets-feminine vibe.

- **BIG, BOLD HOOPS.** These have always looked cooler with flowing hair than with a short do.

- **A KNEE-LENGTH KNIFE-PLEAT SKIRT.** It has the potential to look stuffy, but it telegraphs European chic when paired with messy longer hair (see Lisa and Karen on pages 140–141).

- **CLASSIC BROGUES.** So much more ladylike with an abundant head of hair.

Long hair is a great accessory in its own right. Molly's hair is a huge part of her style. Just check it out: superlong, strong, blond. She would look like an entirely different person if she cut it. I vote she keep her glorious hippie hair *forever*. Her secret is that she takes good care of it.

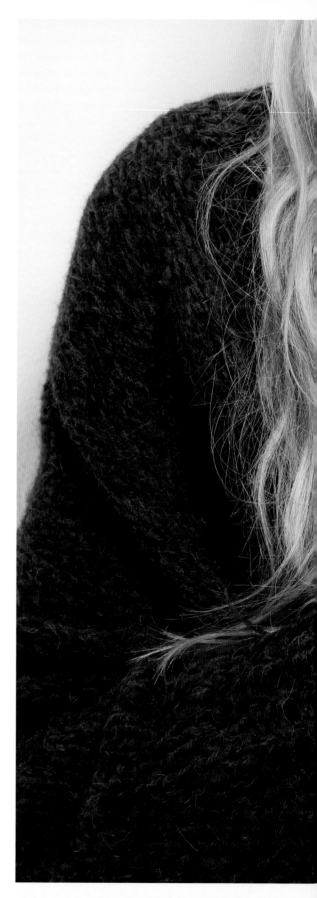

"I highlight every two months or so; my hair grows really fast. I wash it with a mixture of baking soda and apple-cider vinegar (I like ShamPHree, by the How-To Hair Girl) to balance hair and scalp without stripping away the natural oils. It gives me the waves and texture of 'second-day' hair for days!"

—Molly Guy

The Joys of Short Hair

Short hair was *it* in the swinging sixties. Think of Mia Farrow and Twiggy, looking all gamine in their A-line minis, block-heeled Mary Janes, flirty eyelashes—and super-cropped locks. Short dos came back again in a big way in the 1980s and '90s, when models like Esmé Marshall, Linda Evangelista, and Christy Turlington chopped it all off—shedding their girl-next-door prettiness for an edgier stance.

I love short hair on younger girls because it gives them a tomboyish French-waif look. And I love it on older women when done right—that is, not a sensible chop designed to keep the hair out of their eyes, but something deliberate, a little edgy and even a bit sexy.

It definitely takes guts to go this route: with nothing to hide behind, you feel literally exposed. So the cut has to be the right shape for your face, and style is essential.

Jeanine offsets her punky chop with edgy Dior pearl earrings and a frothy lace dress.

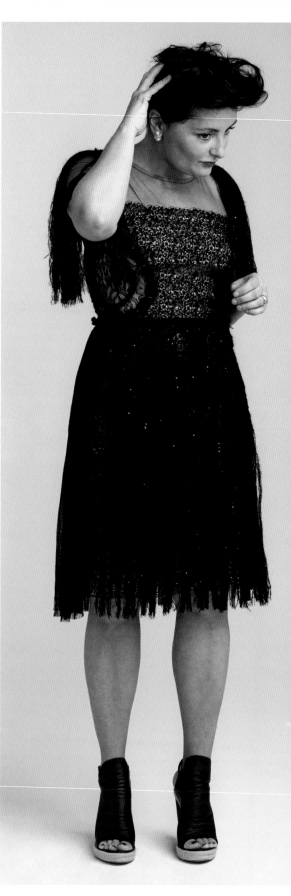

Dressing for Short Hair

Thinking about going short? Take a cue from Meredith, who cut her just-past-the-shoulders hair super short a few years ago. Ever since then, she has been experimenting with makeup and often sports red lipstick or bolder eye shadow. You can also get away with wearing big earrings like chandelier drops; set against shorter locks, they look more gamine and less bohemian.

What Works with Short Hair

- Turtlenecks

- High-neck or bow blouses

- Plunging necklines (or backs)

- Big, dangling earrings (not hoops)

For a Girl-Meets-Boy Vibe

- Floral prints

- Long skirts (which can look too frumpy on longer-haired women)

- Pencil skirts

- Anything lacy but not overly frilly

- Sexy, strappy, pointy-toed heels

"I cut my hair short because I never had a good hairstyle: it was neither here nor there. So I mostly wore a ponytail, which felt lame. Cutting it has been liberating: I spend less time on my hair, it looks more 'done,' and it's awesome in the summer. Since my haircut, I've been weirdly focused on getting my nails done and wearing more eye makeup and fancier or higher-heeled shoes to offset the boyishness."

—Meredith Rollins

Hair Color Can Change Your Life

The right subtle color brightens your face and takes years off your appearance. Before I go on about my own hair color exploits, I want to tell the story of my good friend Liz, a very cool chick who at one point in her life did not have a cool-chick hair color: it was too ashy, when what she needed was warm highlights. And one day, I just had to tell her: "You're cool and you dress cool . . . but your hair color is *not* cool." And yes, we're still friends. In fact, she went straight to the salon and got proper beachy strands and thanked me profusely.

As for my own color: my naturally dark hair sometimes looks too harsh for my skin tone—a common phenomenon as we get older. Luckily, I found Tracey Cunningham, inventor of the ombré trend and one of L.A.'s most sought-after colorists—I've sat next to everyone from Charlize Theron to Gwyneth Paltrow in her salon, Mèche.

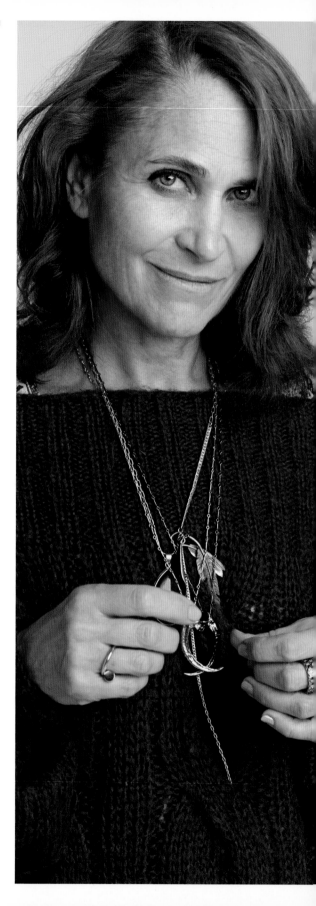

BOLD MOVES. When it comes to color, sometimes it's better to think outside the box. While not everyone can pull off cool blue hair like Susan's, there are tons of new shades—from light lavender to pale yellow—to give you a little edge.

"Years ago, I spied a gorgeous and very sophisticated older woman with hair tinted a superchic steel blue. I thought, *This is the way to go when the time is right for a major change!* Last year, I got to that point where dark hair was too much but I wasn't ready to go gray: it's so aging to my eyes. A faded denim hue was *my* way to go."

—Susan Houser

Q&A with Tracey Cunningham

What do you recommend to someone who wants a change but has never colored her hair?

I often start with fine highlights plus a gloss to give them a taste. An allover single process would ruin the hair. Less is more!

How can someone know what color is right for her?

Schedule a consultation, and don't rush it. I can suggest a particular color that suits your skin and eyes, but you may envision something totally different. Be sure to account for makeup and style; if you're good with makeup, any hair color can look amazing on you.

How can you avoid damaging your hair?

By going to a colorist who is careful. Also, Olaplex—a professional product developed to protect hair and prevent breakage—has transformed the art of hair coloring, allowing us to push the envelope so much further. I feel like it gives me superpowers!

What kind of highlights should you ask for: Balayage [random hand-painted streaks]? Foil?

Either is fine—as long as you have a good person doing it. Go to someone who's the best at what she does. Don't ask a balayage specialist for foils.

Gray Hair: Hide It or Flaunt It?

More women these days are eschewing the hair-color roller coaster and gracefully going gray. But this is no easy feat. From growing out your roots to homing in on the right shade of gray, the process can be harrowing. Thankfully, Dana Ionato has all the answers. A top colorist at Sally Hershberger in New York, she is the vision behind some of the most fashionable heads in town.

Q&A with Dana Ionato

How do you go from coloring your hair to going gray—and avoid that awkward skunk phase?

The less color, the better—especially with ammonia-based products. You can stop touching up the roots and low-light only where grays start showing, strategically placing your natural color around the hairline and in the part. That eradicates the regrowth line and distracts from the gray. Do this gradually until more of the gray grows out. Stick with one colorist during this phase: bouncing around will not help!

Blondes who highlight and get their roots done should stop and do highlights only, to turn the grays blond. Your hair may look lighter without the added dimension of highlights, so be prepared.

For redheads and brunettes, if you're only about 25 percent gray, have your stylist use low-lights that only cover the unwanted silvery bits. It makes the root look less crazy but doesn't oversaturate hair. Just let the root grow out and keep cutting the ends.

Why is removing color from already-colored hair *not* the solution?

The bottom will never match the top, and the process lifts off the pigments. This is a very aggressive and damaging procedure that will not result in a natural salt-and-pepper gray: it will lift to an icy silver blond that looks like a platinum double process. If you're lucky enough to have mostly white hair—not salt and pepper—then you'll have an easier time of lifting it all to a solid white.

Is growing in one's gray an option for everyone?

We all have different variations of salt and pepper in our hair; some ladies don't have enough white to achieve the effect. I treat each client differently depending on her hair texture and gray percentage. It's up to the client how much she will sacrifice, and if she is willing to stick to the plan. Less hair color is necessary for the most dramatic result. It's a waiting game that most people don't have the patience for.

People think they want to stop coloring their hair and go gray, but they often hate the outcome. Gray hair is the absence of pigment; without pigment in your hair, more makeup will be required to enhance your natural features.

How do you prevent brassy undertones—and the spray-painted look—if you dye your hair brown?

Once you start covering grays, the problem becomes getting the brown to match your natural hair without looking too dark or dyed. The colorist must use the right product and formula for your percentage of gray.

I start all clients with semi-permanent hair color, which looks more natural. It blends the gray, is a little more translucent than permanent color, and fades as you wash it. This way, they can get an idea of what maintenance will be required. Too often, gray coverage—especially for brunettes—starts to darken from buildup. Ask for a half-shade lighter in your hairline. It's a headache for the colorist, but you will achieve much more natural results. The driest, most porous hair that's in the hairline "grabs" the dark, opaque color faster. Be sure that the colorist applies the color neatly and doesn't overlap it, which is what creates buildup—and thus the spray-painted effect.

I always recommend an opalescent gloss to add shine and layer in violet hues to make hair look more vibrant and lustrous.

To make the color last as long as possible?

Use color-safe products! I like Shu Uemura, but there are also plenty available at the drug store; L'Oréal Vive Pro is a great line.

Secrets of Age-Defying Hair

"I don't believe in shampooing daily, so I wash my hair only once a week and let it air-dry. Since I color every six weeks, I use a sulfate-free shampoo as well as Carol's Daughter Monoi Oil shampoo and conditioner. And Shu Uemura's nourishing protective oil is fantastic and smells so good. I trim my hair every three months but should probably do it more often."

—Caroline Forsling

Caroline has the epitome of youthful hair.

Only recently did I start to understand the concept of youthful hair—that is, hair that's shiny and bouncy versus frizzy and dull. To achieve it, take advice from Anessa Daviero, owner of New York's Headdress Hair Salon and one of very few people to whom I entrust my locks. She knows hair—how it sits, moves, and reacts—and how to make it look ageless.

Q&A with Anessa Daviero

What's your philosophy on setting your hair up for success at the salon?

I love cutting hair in a way that lets natural texture reveal itself, keeping any layers loose and cut internally. The cowlicks and odd nuances that make hair special come out when it isn't forced into a style. Younger-looking hair is shiny and healthy with natural movement and texture and colors that are almost uneven—perfectly imperfect.

What kinds of products do you recommend using?

A shampoo without any detergents, sulfates, or chemical additives has made the biggest difference in my clients' hair—and my own. Detergent-free cleansers clean your scalp without stripping the natural oils. I also do a monthly conditioning treatment because my hair is long: the longer the hair, the older it is, so it needs more moisture. I love Purely Perfect Cleansing Creme and Rahua's Omega 9 hair mask, which has coconut oil, a natural surfactant.

Anything else we can do to retain that youthful shine?

I highly recommend brushing your hair with natural-bristle brushes by Mason Pearson and Janeke, an Italian line we just started carrying. This is super invigorating and helps move natural oils from your scalp to the ends.

Put Down the Brush!

My version of perfect hair has never been "perfect" hair. It looks much more effortless and chic to let it be, especially when you're dressed up. Take a lesson from the Europeans, who *always* forgo the crazy updos and flawless blowouts in favor of a more devil-may-care bedhead—even on the red carpet at the Cannes Film Festival and at fancy parties.

My hair is wavy and coarse, so I have to be very careful not to overdo anything lest it become a big, wild ball. My latest obsession is Philip B. Russian Amber Imperial Shampoo, which is ridiculously expensive but an anti-aging miracle. I swear my hair has never looked better. I use it once a week with a teensy bit of conditioner, comb it through in the shower, add a few drops of Living Proof Full Thickening Cream and a dab of Rodin hair oil—that's it. Also important is getting a trim at least every six months to keep the dead ends from ruining your overall style.

My friend Anne takes a similarly less-is-more approach to her hair.

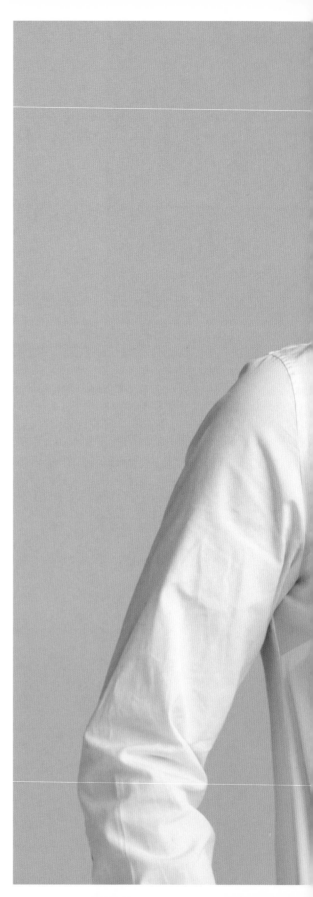

"I don't brush my hair. I only use a wide-tooth comb in the shower after shampooing and conditioning. I like it to look undone, so I mess up my part and tease it with my fingers throughout the day. When putting it up in a half-looped ponytail, I pull it back with my fingers to make sure it's not too perfect. I've recently discovered the wonders of going to the salon for a little keratin treatment to get rid of frizz and make my hair hang the way I've always wanted it to. Caveat: *never* get the heavy-duty version of the treatment, which makes your hair look like a limp broom, and only go to someone with a great track record."

—Anne Johnston Albert

Embrace Your Waves

Naturally curly or wavy hair is way better than a severe blowout, which to me reads conventional and boring. If you're blessed with something as cool as curls, why fight them?

"My hair, for better or worse, has been my trademark forever—it's the first thing people notice and comment on. I've always worn it curly, but the length has gone up and down. (My '80s bob was not a good look!) I didn't start highlighting my hair until my thirties, though. I was a real blonde until my twenties, but my hair darkened as I got older and spent less time in the sun. Now I'm the blondest I've been since my teens—it helps camouflage the encroaching grays!"
—Susan Kaufman

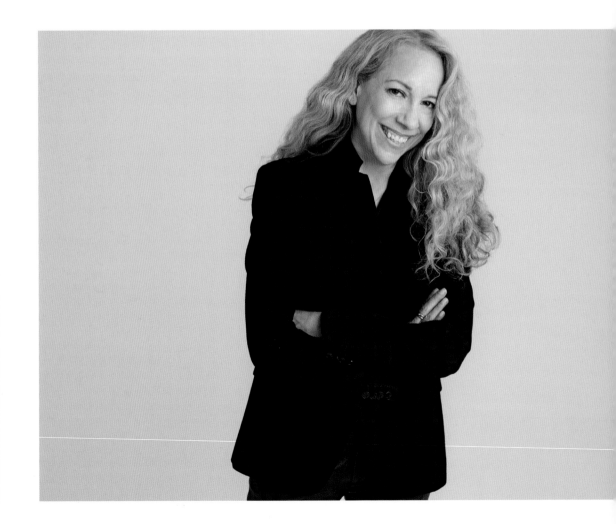

STAYING NATURAL. Brooke has amazingly full hair—but that wasn't always the case, as she caved to societal pressure and straightened it for many years. Thankfully, she came to her senses and now lets her natural beauty shine through.

"Crucial to healthy hair is a good cut—the best you can afford. I get my hair cut only once a year, but the cut is so great that it grows out nicely and holds its shape. I've gone to April Barton at Suite 303 in New York for thirteen years; she cut my hair for my wedding and I never looked back."

—Brooke Williams

The Right Skin and Makeup Routines Are Key

Looking effortlessly cool isn't just about the proper mix of clothes and attitude. It's also about how you put your face and hair together. Too much makeup is never a good idea, and overdone hair and nails feel too, well, overdone. I, as well as all the women in this book, are proponents of natural beauty—of highlighting the aspects of your appearance that you love, not covering up those you don't like. Don't get me wrong: I use a mix of Josie Maran tinted moisturizer and her Argan Illuminizer with a drop of Bobbi Brown bronzing gel and a dusting of Guerlain's Terracotta bronzer to make my skin look as vibrant as possible. The trick is knowing when enough is enough.

"I don't use much makeup, but I am particular about my skin. I scrub it three times a week and massage it daily with a few drops of amazing Odielle Rose Serum by my friend makeup artist Marie-Josée Leduc, which leaves my skin smooth and hydrated. When I do wear makeup, I like it to be invisible—nude colors that match my complexion for smooth-looking skin. Then I finish with a dusting of Golden Baked Powder by Black Radiance on the apples of my cheeks, bridge of my nose, and tip of my chin and collarbones. Instant luminosity guaranteed!"
—Pascale Poma

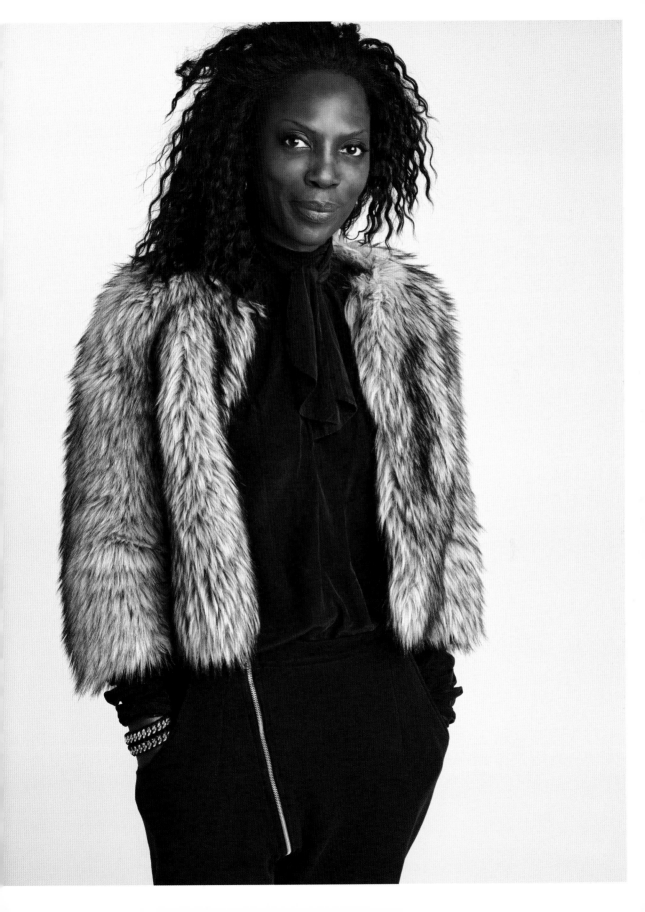

Q&A with Molly Guy, Founder of Stone Fox Bride

What was your first fashion splurge and why?

In 1986, I was walking home from my best friend Josie's house and spotted a wet twenty-dollar bill on the ground. The next day I marched to the mall after school and bought a floppy red wool hat with a black bow at the Limited Express that cost $19.99. As a third grader, being able to channel my inner Anita Pallenberg and saunter through the hallways of my Chicago public school, Newberry Academy, in a bright red floppy hat with a black bow from the Limited made me feel positively rock star-worthy. I went from being a geek with blue glasses and braces who owned a turtle to a bona fide rock star's wife.

Who are your style icons?

I think of my friend Aliza, for some reason. I've known her since grade school, and she just has the most perfect, awesome, understated style. She lives in Silver Lake with her two kids and husband, Lance, and is the most mellow, easygoing person ever. She has an amazing eye and is a genius at thrifting. Everything she owns she's thrifted from the tiniest little Salvation Army stores all over the country. I don't think she's ever spent more than forty dollars on one item. Her clothes and furniture are super pristine, perfect, bohemian, and high-end. There is a running mantra in my head: "WAA?" (Would Aliza approve?)

What are your go-to jeans? How do you usually style them?

I love a good skinny jean, slightly cropped, that I cut at the hem with my daughter's crafts scissors.

Go-to weekend outfit?

Isabel Marant boots, skinny jeans, old black tee, black Ryan Roche sweater, thrifted Stella McCartney cape over a black leather jacket.

What did you used to wear all the time that you wouldn't dream of wearing now?

Seven jeans with a thong, a padded bra, and a fitted Only Hearts see-through lingerie tank with false eyelashes and hair extensions (don't ask—weird phase when I was twenty-five).

Foolproof evening or party look?

I'm a working mom who goes to bed super early, so it would have to be a mask of full-fat Greek yogurt and my grandpa Sol's nightshirt from the '60s.

Any signature beauty or hair thing you do?

I've slept in braids every night for the past six years. Great for my waves, bad for my sex life.

Any length and fit rules you do or don't follow?

I love a good muumuu.

Do you only have expensive designer clothing or do you mix?

I don't care about labels . . . some of my best pieces are ones that I've thrifted or gotten at garage sales that are totally anonymous.

Name five things you think every woman should have in her closet.

A cozy sweater; jeans that make her feel like a million bucks; beat-up, worn black boots; a tattered sexy lingerie slip for sleeping or for wearing on late summer nights spent at an outdoor party with strappy sandals and too much blue eyeliner; a signature fragrance.

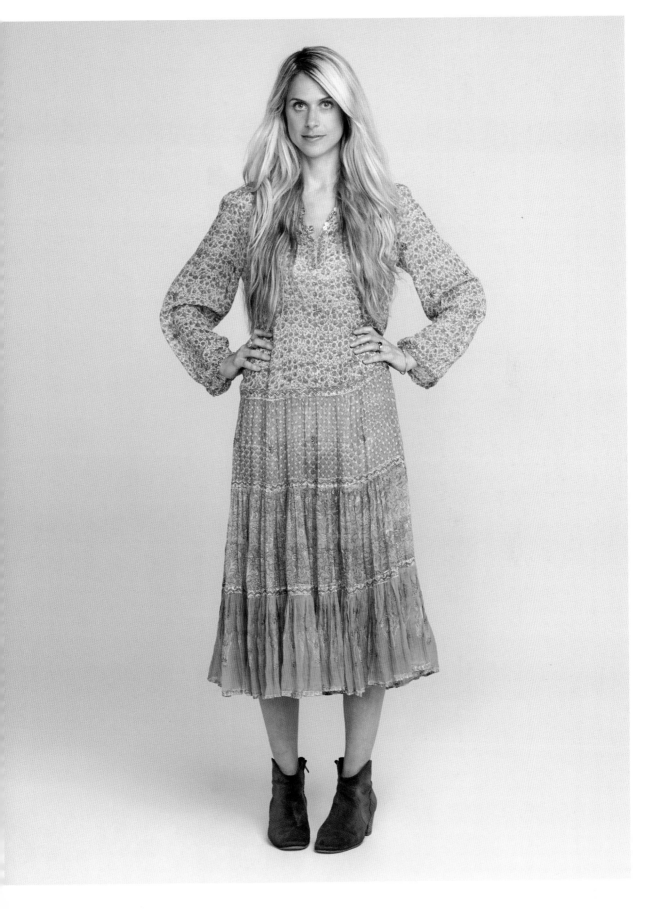

IF IT DOESN'T FIT, IT'S NOT COOL

How a garment drapes on your body is just as important as its fabric, design, and construction quality. An ill-fitting piece— whether too big or too snug—will *never* look good on you, no matter how beautiful it is. More to the point, it has to fit right for what it is. Baggy pieces need to be the *right* kind of baggy; same goes for tight or fitted garments.

How many times have you bought something because you just *had* to have it, even though it didn't fit properly? You might love something on the hanger—a moleskin jacket, say—but when you try it on, the shoulders are wrong or it hits too low on your leg or hip. Don't despair: you needn't forgo such items if you know how to fix them. Learn the miracles that are tailoring and shoe repair, and become a master customizer.

I certainly have. Over the years, I've taken many things—jeans, army jackets, sweaters—to my tailor and dramatically transformed them into go-to pieces. If your favorite pair of jeans suddenly feels wrong because they're too wide at the bottom, take them in a bit and maybe crop them, and voilà: a whole new pair of pants. Think of it as shopping in your own closet—with a little help from your trusty tailor.

Fit Clinic

Skirts

Think of these as a really feminine pants alternative: a ladylike or boho "bottom" instead of jeans or trousers. Depending on the top you pair them with, you can create lots of different looks.

PENCIL AND A-LINE SKIRTS should be knee-length—meaning they can hit anywhere from the top to the bottom of your kneecap; the choice is yours. (Anything higher can get tricky unless you have supermodel legs or ones that you love to show off.)

MIDI LENGTH is a hard one unless you really adore your legs: midis often hit at the largest part of the calf but are more flattering if the hem falls just above that point, showing off the taper of the muscle.

MAXI SKIRTS should almost but not quite sweep the floor. Otherwise they can look dorky or awkwardly bell-like instead of fluid and dramatic.

Pants

My favorite bottoms are pants—all kinds, from jeans to menswear trousers. I just feel like I can achieve anything in the right pair (plus they're supercomfortable!).

WIDE-LEG TROUSERS look best when they almost completely cover your shoes—like Anna's on page 39. This way, you achieve the lengthiest leg possible with an added element of slouchy cool.

JEANS can work a number of ways, from hitting just above the ankle bone (great for summer) to a cute straight-leg that fits snugly around the ankle. A length that hits just at the top of the foot is most versatile. If the jeans are flared, I advise a more generous length (see wide-leg trousers, above), or a kicky crop.

STRAIGHT-LEG SUIT PANTS are good at ankle length or just below the ankle. Alternatively, they can have a nice "break" right at your shoe.

Does Size Really Matter?

Too many of us worry about what number (0 to 14 and up) or letter (XS to XL) we are. Ignore the manufacturer's label and go with what actually looks right on your body. So many American lines fake their sizes anyway. For instance, J. Crew sometimes offers XXXS, which is really just a European extra-small. I know an independent designer who switched the labels in her skinny pants from 6 to 4 just so more women would buy them (and they did). Pretty silly, right? Go with what fits, what looks right, and what's most comfortable on *you.*

Quick Fixes

Reinvent Old Faves

Do you have pieces lurking in the back of your closet that you love but never wear? Don't throw them out; remake them! But be sure to enlist the aid of a reputable tailor and make him or her your best friend.

MAXI COATS. A simple hem is all it takes to transform an overlong design into a knee-length, pea, or car coat (which should hit a few inches below the waist).

PADDED-SHOULDER BLAZERS. Swap too-big shoulder pads for a smaller size and have a tailor nip in the center-back seam a smidge.

SHAPELESS OVERSIZE SWEATERS. Slimmify the arms slightly (ask the tailor to sew a new seam) for a slouchy-chic (versus baggy) silhouette. This applies only to machine-made tight knits.

LONG EVENING DRESSES. Shorten to a cool midi length or reinvent as a little cocktail dress.

SHIRTDRESSES. Give these a new lease on life by hemming them into long, slightly butt-skimming shirts.

LONG SLIPS. Convert them into camisoles, which you can wear myriad ways. Don't be afraid to chop them yourself and leave the edges raw.

HANDBAGS. If the strap is too short or too long, head to your shoemaker, who can make a simple alteration for you.

Tailoring Tips: Pants

Don't blow off buying a pair of pants if you really love them but they're not a perfect fit. Your tailor can take them from so-so to stellar with just a few quick fixes.

- **IF YOU HAVE STOVEPIPE PANTS** (i.e., legs the same width from top to bottom), taper them only slightly—a half inch or so—from the mid-knee down. This gives the body a slimmer look. But don't peg them too much or you'll end up with jodhpurs.

- **IF YOU HAVE SLIGHT SADDLEBAGS**, take in the outer-thigh area just a bit, right where the offending bags are, so the pant leg is super straight. This nip and tuck is like a visual Spanx, fooling the eye into seeing a leaner silhouette.

- **IF YOU'RE TALL AND CAN NEVER FIND LONG-ENOUGH JEANS**, have a tailor stitch a denim piece at the bottom. This solution looks especially cool when the denim hues don't quite match.

- **IF YOUR SKINNY PANTS BUNCH AT THE ANKLE**, have the seam opened just enough so the hem fits over your shoes. Lately, I prefer opening the inside seam of the pant leg, because it looks fresher (and is less noticeable).

Tailoring Tip: Button-Downs

I love everything about a crisp cotton button-down—except how the placket buckles between the buttons to reveal skin underneath. So sloppy! So, since I never wear my shirts opened all the way, I get the placket sewn from a few buttons down—wherever I want to start showing skin. It still looks like a normal button-down (but you put it on over your head, like a T-shirt), but you get no peekaboo skin. Pretty genius, if I do say so myself! Note: run the stitch down the inside of the button line for the most natural look.

Almost Always Needs a Tweak: The Jumpsuit

Love a jumpsuit but can't find one that fits correctly? Same here. I'm pretty short—only five feet three inches—so the crotch never hits where it should. It seems like an ordeal, but a tailor can move the waistband so the piece fits you better everywhere. Knees on jumpsuits are often a problem for me, too; they usually need to be slightly narrowed. Note that these same guidelines apply to overalls, should you be into them.

Fit Math

It's All About Proportion

Now that you know how individual pieces should fit—and how they can be customized to fit even better—here's a secret: balanced proportions are just as important. Always look at your outfit as a whole: top and bottom should work in concert to create a pleasing silhouette—what I call the big/skinny ratio. Your skinny jeans fit great in the seat and on the leg—but what shape shirt or sweater do you pair with them? The answer is not something equally slim. Tight with tight tends to read tacky. Opt instead for a loose, blousy top, a drapey tee, or a boxy sweater.

A Quick Body Ratio Guide

Make "big/skinny" your mantra; your eye will adjust.

IF YOU'RE . . .	THEN . . .
TOP-HEAVY	Opt for an open neckline, which creates visual white space. Covering up can have the opposite effect, making you look bigger
PEAR-SHAPED	Surprise! Skinnier pants and skirts will look better on you. Why? Because going the "cover-up" route with oversize pieces makes you look dumpy. Showing your curves is much more flattering.
THICK IN THE MIDDLE	Accentuate your lower half with something slim and high-waisted, which will conceal and minimize your middle while flaunting your legs to best effect.
LONG-WAISTED	A higher-waist bottom will create the illusion of lengthier legs. Steer clear of short jackets, which will make your waist look even longer.
SHORT-WAISTED	Go for low-rise cuts, which will hit just right on your body. Don't tuck in too-bulky tops or you'll look like a cinched paper bag.

5 Things That Should Fit Big

1. PARKAS. Not only does oversize look cooler, it also lets you add more layers underneath.

2. CHINOS. They should have just the right amount of slouch: big enough that you need a belt to keep them up. You can cinch them or wear them a bit low on your hips.

3. BOYFRIEND BLAZERS. These should fit in the shoulders but can otherwise be boxy and a bit overlong. Have a tailor shorten the sleeves so you don't look like a little girl in her dad's coat. (Or you can just scrunch them up, but avoid rolling them, which looks sloppy and too specifically '80s.)

4. DENIM CUTOFFS. Shorts are much more flattering when there's a little room around the thigh.

5. MENSWEAR CARDIGANS. Exaggerated sizing is the whole point, right?

5 Things That Should Fit Small

1. ANKLE BOOTS. These should be snug around the ankle, creating a nice silhouette with a cropped pant.

2. CARDIGANS FOR LAYERING. I like to wear a formfitting cardie under a big one when it's really cold outside—for chic *and* warmth.

3. LONG TANKS. Great to wear under sheer pieces. The closer to the body the better, so you don't compromise the shape of the shirt or sweater you're wearing over it.

4. SKINNY JEANS. While they shouldn't be so tight that they look like leggings or sausage casings, they *are* meant to be skinny.

5. T-SHIRTS. The ones that you wear with baggier bottoms should fit snugly (not tight).

Shoe Fit

Don't Neglect Your Beloved Shoes

I make a habit of stopping by my favorite shoe guy Erik's shop (on Grand and Essex in New York City, if you're ever in that neighborhood) every time I buy a new pair. The first thing I do is have him put a protective layer of thin rubber on the bottom, which (a) makes them a bit more comfortable for walking on cement sidewalks and (b) prolongs their life by a mile. Find a shoe guy you can trust who gets you—and what you like. He can perform the following magic tricks.

- **MAKE IT POSSIBLE FOR YOU TO WALK IN THOSE HEELS.** Whenever I buy shoes that prove too high to walk in normally, Erik cuts just a little off the heel, making sure not to ruin the pitch of the shoe. (The maximum amount will depend on the shoe design.) Even a quarter of an inch makes a difference without sacrificing the look. Nothing is less cool than teetering in your too-tall shoes.

- **CHANGE THE COLOR.** Love the shoes, hate the hue? Don't ditch them; dye them black. It's one of the easiest alterations for a cobbler to execute and it's like getting a whole new pair of shoes. Black is pretty hard to mess up, but don't try this with crazy colors (although I did turn a pair of boots an amazing metallic silver once).

- **CREATE "NEW" SHOES FOR LESS THAN THIRTY DOLLARS.** Own a pair of knee-high boots that you love but never wear? Have your shoemaker chop off the top to make cute ankle boots. But first, determine *exactly* where you want them to hit on your leg; do this while trying them on, not by just eyeing them.

- **GIVE SHOES A LONGER LIFE.** Always bring new leather-soled shoes straight to your repair guy like I do—prior to wearing them out for the first time—to apply thin rubber pads on the sole. This increases the cushioning and protects the shoe. If Erik recommends it, I'll add taps to the heels, too. And pay attention: as soon as a heel wears down, have it fixed. Shabby-looking shoes can completely undermine an otherwise put-together outfit. Don't be afraid to chop them yourself and leave the edges raw.

The Right Shoes Can Make You Look Thinner

You will never see me in ladylike pumps or dainty sandals, and here's why: given my body's proportions, they make me seem heavier than I am. The tinier your foot looks, the bigger the rest of your body will appear in comparison. (I call this Small-Foot Syndrome.) For some reason, this most applies when I'm wearing jeans. I always opt for a substantial shoe like chunky yet refined boots, clogs, or platforms, which creates a stronger anchor and fools the eye into seeing a sleeker silhouette.

Q&A with Lisa Immordino Vreeland, Filmmaker

Who are your style icons?

I have always been inspired by Marchesa Casati's style and her life.

What are the items in your closet that you've had the longest and will never throw out?

I can easily say that two pairs of Prada boots will go down in history as the oldest boots ever owned.

Name some fashion rules you live by.

Ironed T-shirts—since I dress so casually, an ironed T-shirt makes it look all spruced up.

Great jewelry—I love Ten Thousand Things and wear multiple necklaces at once.

Great posture—everything looks bad on people who do not hold themselves well.

Personal style—wear what you are comfortable in; do not be a victim of the fashion moment.

What are your go-to jeans? How do you usually style them?

Jeans have to be only in white for me. I remember that I did not allow my daughter, Olivia, to wear any blue jeans until she was eight years old. She was so happy that she slept in them the first night.

What are your favorite accessories?

A nice leather bag and shawls.

Is there anything you do that breaks conventional fashion rules?

I am so conventional but very *"bien dans ma peau."*

Any good styling tricks? Belting, layering, rolling, cropping?

I love cooking, so I normally have my sleeves rolled up (so I don't get anything on them). I sometimes forget to pull them down, so now it's my "thing."

Do you only have expensive designer clothing or do you mix?

I am a big believer in mixing labels and really do not focus on them. Quality is what counts.

Do you have any fashion pet peeves?

I personally do not wear patterns, so I am a bit sensitive to it.

Is there anything you've owned and worn for more than fifteen years?

For some reason all of my workout clothes are very old: old Adidas sweatpants, the perfect navy blue Nike running pants, and my brother's old sweatshirts.

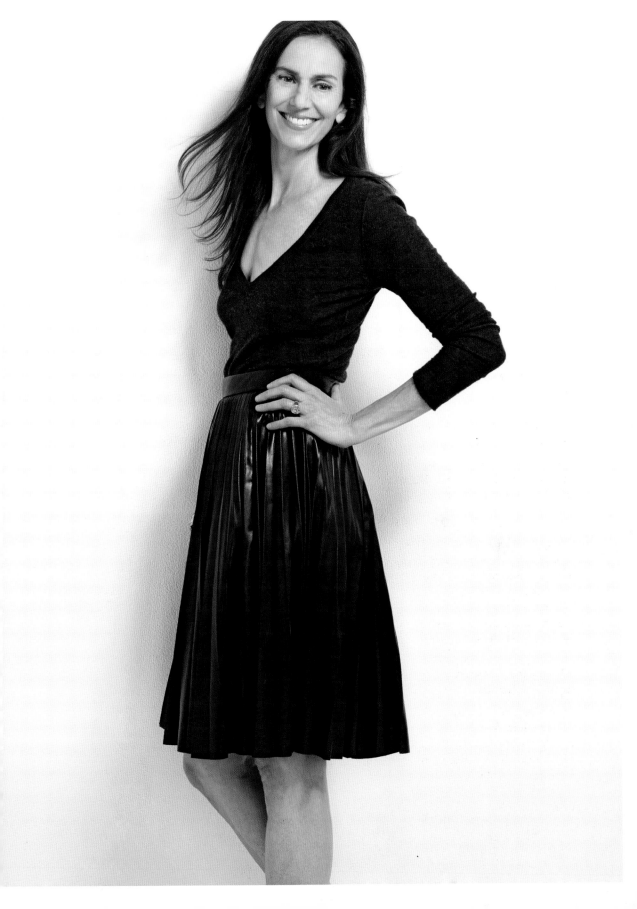

The Cool 20

Here are the staples every woman needs to build her wardrobe. Start with these and add "excitement" pieces from here. Some might be obvious, but others will surprise you.

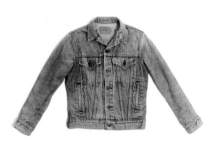

1. CLASSIC DENIM JACKET. For layering—or for wearing on its own.

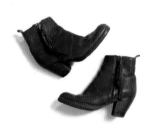

2. WALKABLE ANKLE BOOTS. Either pointy or slightly rounded in the toe. You can wear them with everything from jeans to knee-length skirts.

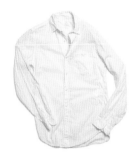

3. OVERSIZE WHITE BUTTON-DOWN. Roll up the sleeves, half tuck it in—everything else you're wearing will look classically cool.

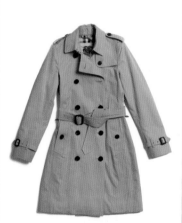

4. TRENCH COAT. Adds instant French mystery.

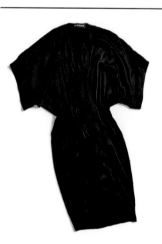

5. SIMPLE BLACK DRESS. Dress it up, dress it down, wear it forever.

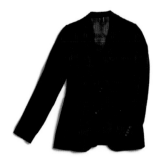

6. BLACK OR NAVY TAILORED BLAZER. Will *never* look old.

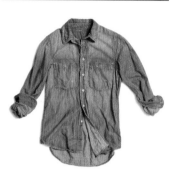

7. DENIM SHIRT. Whether pristine or a bit ripped and frayed, it will add a slight toughness under blazers.

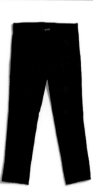

8. MEN'S-STYLE TROUSERS. Slouchy or fitted, they are a great work staple (and, with a plain tee, a nice jeans alternative).

9. CHUNKY MENSWEAR WATCH. Looks rich and slightly European.

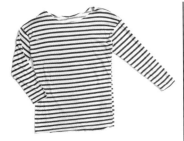

10. STRIPED SAILOR SHIRT. For a cute French look.

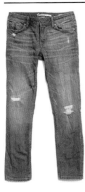

11. CLASSIC FIVE-POCKET JEANS. This staple can be worn so many ways.

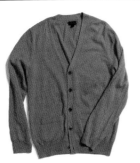

12. MEN'S-STYLE CARDIGAN. The perfect cozy layer.

13. SMALL "ESSENTIALS" BAG. Great to tuck into your tote or to carry around solo on the weekends when your load is lighter.

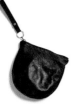

14. MEN'S-STYLE VEST. Layer it under a big cardigan or blazer to add interest.

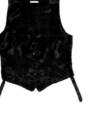

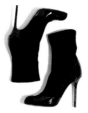

15. SEXY ANKLE BOOTS. Ditto, but also appropriate for evening: try them in place of fancy heels.

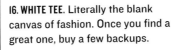

16. WHITE TEE. Literally the blank canvas of fashion. Once you find a great one, buy a few backups.

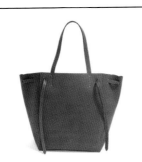

17. ROOMY LEATHER TOTE. A must-have for work.

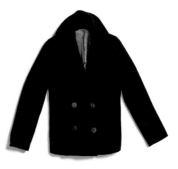

18. PEACOAT. Choose one with military edge or that's superclean and classic, depending on what you plan to pair it with.

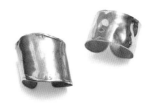

19. BOLD CUFF. Adds drama to anything.

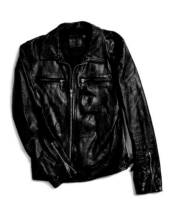

20. CLASSIC BIKER JACKET. Because nothing will make you feel cooler!

10 Rules to Live By

1. DON'T SETTLE ON JUST OK OR YOU'LL HAVE A WHOLE CLOSETFUL OF "JUST OKS." If you're on the hunt for the perfect pair of whatever—black pants, white jeans, brown ankle boots in the "right" brown—don't buy them unless you really think they're perfect. I can't tell you how many times I've looked for something specific and found the "almost good enough" version and bought it. Then I found another that was a little better than the first and bought that one. And then another. You see where I'm going with this. I ended up with way too many "almost good" pieces. **Either wait until you find the right one or get something that you can turn into the perfect piece at the tailor or shoemaker.**

2. THROW OUT THINGS THAT DON'T SPEAK TO YOU. This is one I'm stealing from Japanese clutter guru Marie Kondo. She's way more spiritual about this than I am (she thinks clothes have feelings), but really pay attention to what's in your drawers and closet. **If you pick something up and you don't love it, donate it or give it to a friend.**

3. DON'T FANTASY SHOP. I used to do this more when I was younger, but no one is immune, and it goes a little something like this:

You're shopping on a random day, just for sport. In other words, you're not looking for anything in particular—you are not on the hunt for a waterproof jacket, say. So you're hanging with a friend and shop-hopping. You spot an ankle-length crocheted dress with bell sleeves and you immediately *have* to have it.

You: "Look at this gorgeous thing! I have to try it on."

Friend: "Um . . . yeah, it's super cool, but where would you wear it?"

You: "What do you mean?! I will wear it when . . . when . . . I will wear it when I'm dancing on a misty mountaintop with Robert Plant!"

Friend: "Put it back."

This sounds funny, but it happens to the best of us. So while none of us really think we're going to be hanging out with Robert Plant back in the '70s anytime soon, we do have the ability to make excuses and fake occasions to justify purchases. I've heard them all, from "I will wear this on fancy dates" to "I need this for when I get my arms super fit." If you're someone who is most comfortable in jeans, boots, and tees, you will probably *never* find yourself in need of a black sequined car coat or a pair of four-inch strappy heels. If you're not shopping for a specific fancy occasion, skip it. Just remember who you are and what works best for you. **If something doesn't fit into your lifestyle, you will probably never, ever wear it. Spend your money on what you know you will wear.**

4. DON'T BUY SOMETHING JUST BECAUSE IT'S ON SALE. I have fallen into this trap at sample sales so many times, so trust me on this one! What happens is you get overwhelmed at the idea of the bargain—I once saw a Comme des Garçons brown chiffon tail jacket at one of these events and bought it simply because "Look! I got a Comme des Garçons jacket for $150!" It sat in my closet untouched for years until I gave it to Goodwill. I wouldn't have pined over that thing at its full $1,500 price, so why fawn all over it just because it was within my reach? **The best feeling of all, however, is finding that thing you'd been dying for all season in your size at 50 percent off. Wait for that moment or forget about it.**

5. IF YOU BUY SOMETHING TRENDY, HANG ON TO IT FOR A YEAR BEFORE WEARING IT. And I'm not talking about something so au courant that you need to wear it ASAP or you'll look passé the next year. I mean certain really great pieces that could potentially be ubiquitous, like the amazing satin jacket with an embroidered dragon on the back that I got at Zara. This is a forever piece that needed to sit back awhile until the hype was over. Then when I finally did rock it, it felt brand-new. This also happened with a cute multicolored striped preppie sweater from Gap about twenty years ago. I wanted it so badly but didn't want to wear it during the time it came out. I kept it a while and sprung it out the following season. It might be hard to do, but it really makes you feel like you've got a whole new look once you start wearing it. **Think of this as style insurance.**

6. DON'T WORRY ABOUT DRESSING YOUR AGE! Sure, there are those things you'd wear every week in maximum rotation for like a whole year. Then one day, without warning, you look in the mirror and feel all wrong. I call this the mutton-dressed-as-lamb syndrome, or "Route 66," which is a reference to a woman who was wearing a denim jacket with patches that said "Yield," "Stop," and "Route 66" all over it. From behind, she looked about twenty-three, but when she turned around, I saw that she was surely in her sixties. I have dubbed inappropriate dressing "Route 66" ever since. **But if you have classics that you really love, by all means wear them forever.** This includes denim and leather jackets, jeans, and yes, even overalls. When in doubt, think of Georgia O'Keeffe and how she rocked her twisted classics well into her eighties. Just beware of the manufactured Route 66 pieces that are meant for the kids.

7. SHOP YOUR CLOSET. Sometimes I fall into a fashion rut and after wearing the same thing and feeling great for months, suddenly it feels boring or all wrong. I simply look around my closet and find the polar opposite (like a pretty flowy top after rocking a plain tee all season) and suddenly it all feels fresh again! **Instead of running out to buy more more more, look at your inventory. You might just be surprised.**

8. ALWAYS KEEP THEM GUESSING. In other words, don't fall into the overdone or matchy-matchy trap. Keep things unexpected! Wear a cool old tee under a structured blazer, Birkenstocks with good trousers, or a big ethnic cuff with an evening dress. **When in doubt, mix it up for maximum coolness.**

9. FIND YOUR SIGNATURE PIECE. If you love a white tee, have that be your thing, even when dressed up with a black satin pencil skirt and heels. **If you love jewelry, make a certain piece your everyday item.** This might just come naturally to you because something might have sentimental meaning or just make you feel good and like no one but yourself, which brings me to . . .

10. MOST OF ALL, *BE YOURSELF.* If you really and truly feel like something is "not you" or doesn't fit into your lifestyle, then don't force it. **When something feels right, it shows, and people will look at you and say, "She's really got it!"**

Acknowledgments

It takes many great people to put together a book like this, so I would like to thank the following:

My favorite collaborator—my husband, Michael Waring—who tirelessly shot all of the women in this book and made them look as gorgeous in the photos as they all are in real life; Artisan's Lia Ronnen, who was super gung-ho about this project from day one and whose input and guidance were invaluable every step of the way; my other favorite collaborator, Anne Johnston Albert, my oldest friend and confidante—and guru when it comes to all things style-related—who simultaneously produced the photo shoots and modeled like it was the easiest task in the world (it wasn't); Janeiro Gonzales, one of the most talented makeup artists I've ever worked with, who always makes women look like their best selves (while making them laugh in the process); my brilliant text editor, Jen Renzi, who just got it right away (I will miss our special lunch meetings!); the amazing women at Artisan: Mura Dominko, who was enthusiastic about everything throughout while keeping me on schedule in the nicest possible way, Michelle Ishay-Cohen for making the book look so cool, and Renata Di Biase, Sibylle Kazeroid, and Nancy Murray; my niece Libby Silber for shooting perfect behind-the-scenes photos; my amazing mom, Caryl Linett, a huge style inspiration who's always shown me there was nothing I couldn't do; my friends Liz Kiernan, Kim France, and Hollis Salzman, who patiently listened to me prattle on about everything while I was writing and editing; David Rees and Ronald Anderson for always being supportive and having my back; Sandy Hochheiser for her unwavering support and encouragement; Kristina Pereira Tully and the team at Runner Collective: Tracy, Desiree, and Robin; and of course all of the incredible women who took time out of their insanely busy schedules to participate. Thank you for inspiring me to write this book.

Index

ABOUT THE AUTHOR

Andrea Linett is the founding creative director of *Lucky,* the award-winning magazine about shopping and style. She has held creative director positions at both eBay Fashion and Michael Kors and is the author of *I Want to Be Her!,* a style memoir based on her website of the same name, and coauthor of the bestselling *Lucky Shopping Manual* and *The Lucky Guide to Mastering Any Style.* Linett lives in New York City with her husband, photographer Michael Waring.

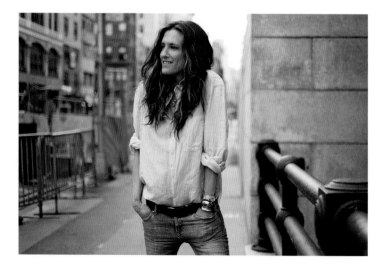